Community-Based Health Organizations

Community-Based Health Organizations

Advocating for Improved Health

Marcia Bayne Smith

Yvonne J. Graham

Sally Guttmacher

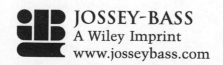

JOSSEY-BASS
A Wiley Imprint
www.josseybass.com

Published by Jossey-Bass
A Wiley Imprint
989 Market Street, San Francisco, CA 94103-1741   www.josseybass.com

Jossey-Bass books and products are available through most bookstores. To contact Jossey-Bass directly call our Customer Care Department within the U.S. at 800-956-7739, outside the U.S. at 317-572-3986 or fax 317-572-4002.

Jossey-Bass also publishes its books in a variety of electronic formats. Some content that appears in print may not be available in electronic books.

Library of Congress Cataloging-in-Publication Data

Bayne Smith, Marcia.
    Community-based health organizations: advocating for improved health/Marcia Bayne Smith, Yvonne Graham, Sally Guttmacher.—1st ed.
       p.; cm.
    Includes bibliographical references and index.
    ISBN 0-7879-6486-7 (alk. paper)
       1. Community health services—United States. 2. Voluntary health agencies—United States. 3. Public health—United States.
       [DNLM: 1. Community Health Services—organization & administration—United States. 2. Voluntary Health Agencies—organization & administration—United States. 3. Vulnerable Populations—United States. WA 546 AA1 B361c 2005] I. Graham, Yvonne, date. II. Guttmacher, Sally. III. Title.
    RA445.B387 2005
    362.1'068—dc22   2004022993

Printed in the United States of America
FIRST EDITION
PB Printing
10 9 8 7 6 5 4 3 2 1

Contents

Tables, Figures, and Exhibits

Tables

Figures

Exhibits

Foreword

Mary E. Northridge

This book is a rallying cry to action for each and every one of us who is concerned about the delivery of health care services to poor and working-class communities anywhere in the United States. The pivotal and long-standing roles the authors have played in the founding and evolution of the Caribbean Women's Health Association (CWHA) in Brooklyn, New York, no doubt provided an inspirational source for the passionate and respectful cores they tapped in writing this hands-on book. The authors voice outrage over the unmet health needs of the largely immigrant and poor populations they serve while dignifying the worth of incorporating the diverse cultural beliefs of people living in underserved communities into the health care delivery systems designed to serve them.

The authors are to be credited with carefully articulating what they mean by community-based health organizations (CBHOs) and how they fit into the current fragmented health care delivery system in the United States. Indeed, CBHOs represent a grassroots effort by marginalized communities to come together to provide essential and humane treatment and prevention services to people who need and desire local, trusted, and culturally competent providers. Despite filling an essential niche for millions of Americans who would have limited or no access to health prevention and treatment services if CBHOs did not currently exist, there is no doubt that the present coverage provided by CBHOs is incomplete and that the continued existence of most CBHOs is precarious. As the authors

Mary E. Northridge, Ph.D., M.P.H., is associate professor of clinical sociomedical sciences at the Mailman School of Public Health, Columbia University, and editor in chief of the *American Journal of Public Health*.

make clear, the ability of a community to organize and advocate for resources is essential to the initial establishment of a CBHO; ensuring its sustainability calls for another set of skills—notably fundraising prowess and financial acumen—that are harder to come by and more difficult to hold on to in the competitive marketplace.

As a result, there is no guarantee that the communities most in need of health care are currently being served by a CBHO or that a CBHO that is fulfilling a vital health care mission will remain financially solvent. Further, given current federal, state, and local policies, the playing field for communities in need is not level, and the rules of the game keep changing. Recent immigrants face extremely unjust barriers in qualifying for, accessing, and benefiting from "mainstream" health care services. Given recent immigration patterns, with increasingly poorer populations who may not be able to speak or write fluent English moving into increasingly underserved urban and rural areas, CBHOs represent a viable, culturally competent model for providing diverse immigrant communities with essential health care and social services that are tailored to their unique needs, backgrounds, and values.

Marcia Bayne Smith, Yvonne J. Graham, and Sally Guttmacher have done their part in drawing from the published literature and reflecting on their own experiences to inform others regarding the effective startup, operation, and sustenance of CBHOs. Notably, they root their book in the history of struggle against oppression and exploitation of people of color and poor and working-class communities to realize their health and well-being through the provision of health and social services that they themselves deem crucial. In addition, although the authors use theory to inform health service delivery—notably the Health Keepers Model developed and used by the Caribbean Women's Health Association—their work is grounded in meeting the immediate health needs of poor and working-class people who are being denied holistic, culturally competent, and affordable health care and prevention services in the wealthiest nation the planet has ever known. Finally, by examining the best practices and lessons learned from their survey of other CBHOs and their firsthand experience with the CWHA, they effectively argue for a key role for CBHOs in meeting the health care needs of marginalized and underserved communities now and in the future.

The rest of us must do our part in ensuring that we move toward a U.S. society where the health needs of everyone are understood and effectively met. For those of us in the academy, this means educating and training students from poor, working-class, and immigrant backgrounds to work in health service delivery as well as in health research, education, and administration; forging interdisciplinary curricula that provide students with a basic understanding of the biomedical and social sciences regarding the determinants of health and the holistic provision of health care; funding student internships and locating student placements in CBHOs, which need and value their skills and are qualified to train and guide them; developing and employing multilevel models to evaluate the effectiveness of programs and interventions designed to improve community health and well-being; and providing scientifically based evidence for policymakers to be used in advocating for the badly needed restructuring of the U.S. health care system and increased funding for establishing and maintaining CBHOs in poor and working-class communities.

If we all do our part in holding our governments accountable for achieving the broader social goals of eliminating disparities in health and health care and in providing vital health and social services to everyone in the United States regardless of the ability to pay, CBHOs would be well positioned to translate these worthy goals into everyday reality. What makes this book so compelling is that the authors write from the insider's perspective of "we" when articulating the health needs of poor and immigrant communities. Organizing and advocacy are essential to ensuring that the rights of disfranchised communities to good health and health care are not ignored. By pulling together, we can realize a new era of hope, civic participation, and caring that will result in more egalitarian, purposeful, and healthy lives for everyone in the United States and in the global society of which we are a part through our shared ancestries and common struggles toward achieving social justice and good health for all.

This book is dedicated to Dr. Marco A. Mason, whose professional work, including his doctoral dissertation, gave life to the idea that the establishment of a community-based health organization, dedicated to improving the health of immigrants and the poor, could become a reality. His scholarly contributions provided the framework for the development of the Caribbean Women's Health Association. His support for its growth throughout the years has been unwavering.

Preface

In February 2002, the Caribbean Women's Health Association, Inc. (CWHA), celebrated twenty years of service to low-income, indigent, and immigrant communities in New York City. In reflecting on the events of those two decades, the evolution, successes, and challenges, several characteristics of community-based health organizations (CBHOs) as a particular genre of health care delivery became clear. First, CBHOs have revived and expanded an old public health approach to the delivery of community health services that offers an alternative to the failing mainstream methods. Many of the strategies and modalities employed by CBHOs, such as the emphasis on outreach, education, and prevention and the use of neighborhood residents as community health workers to facilitate access to care for their fellow community members, are now being used by mainstream organizations. As their role as essential partners in the spectrum of health care delivery becomes more widely recognized, CBHOs are increasingly sought out as partners by mainstream health providers to develop partnerships that will help them provide services.

Those two decades of service also made it clear that most CBHOs are so focused on providing services, advocating for funding, negotiating partnerships to improve community health, and advancing a policy agenda on behalf of their constituents that they often neglect to invest in activities that might build their capacity and help them become more competitive and sustainable. In this observation, the idea for this book was born.

Our aim in this book is to introduce readers, from graduate students to health care providers and from community organizers to research investigators, to CBHOs as viable health delivery alternatives with the potential to improve health outcomes in communities that bear the heaviest burden of health disparities. To accomplish this goal, we provide a historical context as well as some theoretical perspectives that explain the origins and functions of CBHOs. A report on the internal and external activities of a sample of CBHOs from across the United States and a comprehensive case study of one CBHO are also included as groundwork on which researchers can build their own investigations. The information on the political and economic environment is critical, as politics and economics are constantly changing and influence how policies are developed and reformed. Changes in the economic climate also affect the ability of CBHOs to provide services. The chapter on sustainability of CBHOs is intended for all students of community health and provides some critical capacity-building tools for future positioning.

The book is organized into three parts. The introductory chapters in Part One provide a historical overview of community-based organizations and the determinants of community health and highlight both established and emerging theories about the development and growth of CBHOs. Chapter One starts with working definitions of the community-based organizations, advocacy, and community organizing concepts such as social capital, social cohesion, and civil society. It then traces the historical development of community health services from antiquity to the present and also looks at the organizational framework and major structural aspects of CBHOs. Chapter Two uses a variety of theoretical paradigms to explore and explain the viability of CBHOs in organizing and building social capital and cohesion by using adult education methods that lead to empowered communities. The chapters in Part One provide historic, organizational, and theoretical evidence of the contributions of CBHOs toward improving health outcomes in their communities.

Part Two consists of two chapters that closely examine the internal and external operations of CBHOs. Chapter Three analyzes responses to a survey questionnaire and results of six in-depth interviews by examining internal tools such as mission statements, budgets, and clients served. The CBHO study reported in Chapter Three documents the importance of community participation in program planning and advocacy efforts for CBHOs. The study also provides some information on external operations in terms of relationships between the CBHO and other providers, other CBHOs, and funding sources. It also provides some preliminary information on how participating CBHOs emerged, evolved, and sustain their operations and plan for the future. Chapter Four provides a comprehensive analysis of the Caribbean Women's Health Association. It lays out the systems and structures that were put in place as well as the methods and strategies used and the management decisions made to enhance organizational capability and increase program resources to respond to community needs.

Part Three contains three chapters that are vital to understanding the ongoing operations and future of CBHOs. Chapter Five provides a thorough discussion of the political and economic environment in which many CBHOs function. It traces the emergence of power in the city and the strategies needed to harness local resources to provide services for poor communities. It also prescribes a multidisciplinary and multiskilled approach in order to effectively develop and operate CBHOs that are capable of organizing, building, and empowering communities to advocate for improved health. The focus of Chapter Six is on organizational sustainability. It covers the various areas that must be given careful attention, including management information systems, human resources, and fiscal systems, in order to provide strong management and maintain a well-run organization. Chapter Seven presents some promising models and pathways that may provide direction for students, communities, and their partners as they develop services to improve community health.

We hope that this book will guide the work of CBHO managers and administrators, community organizers, community members, providers and other health professionals, mainstream partners, and other stakeholders as they work together to organize, build, and empower communities to advocate for improved health.

November 2004

Marcia Bayne Smith
Laurelton, New York

Yvonne J. Graham
Brooklyn, New York

Sally Guttmacher
New York, New York

Acknowledgments

We are deeply indebted to the founding members, volunteers, and staff of the Caribbean Women's Health Association, who have worked so hard over the years to create an organization that proudly delivers excellent service to our community. We also acknowledge Nehama Teitelman, Ulrika Karlsson, and Savannah Shyne, our research assistants on this book. A huge debt of gratitude is owed to Dr. Ruth Browne, director of the Arthur Ashe Institute for Urban Health at University Hospital of Brooklyn–Downstate Medical Center, who provided staff and resources for the demanding outreach process involved in doing survey research.

The Department of Urban Studies at Queens College, City University of New York, has been particularly instrumental in developing this book project. Special thanks is owed to Dr. Len Rodberg, department chair, whose goodwill and quiet guidance provided strong support for this work. As this is a book about community, we also want to acknowledge colleagues within the Urban Studies Department and the larger Queens College community, especially Dr. Alice Sardell, who provided initial comments and who together with Dr. Tarry Hum, Dr. Madhulika Kandelwahl, and particularly Dr. Cicely Rodway forms a group from whom inspiration and advice are continually drawn.

Last but not least, in a book about community, each of us is indebted to close friends and family. Sally Guttmacher acknowledges the support of her son, Benjamin Holtzman. Yvonne Graham is thankful to Dr. Marco A. Mason, whose guidance and support throughout the years have been consistent and unfailing and who is now charged with taking the CWHA forward as a twenty-first-century organization. Marcia Bayne Smith wishes to acknowledge the support of her husband, Bob; her son and daughter-in-law, Corey and Stacy Smith; her granddaughters, Tori and Jada; her daughter, Tara; and her parents, Herman and Elma Bayne, may they rest in peace.

Community-Based
Health Organizations

The Context of Community-Based Health Organizations (CBHOs)

Part One examines the historical, organizational, and theoretical context of community-based health organizations and their role in advocating for health care. This broad sweep examines societies' efforts to develop organized approaches to address the health needs of their communities through both a historical and a contemporary lens. As a result, the two chapters in this section raise some important questions and attempt to provide some initial answers: What is meant by community health? Why examine CBHOs, and more specifically, why study the advocacy function of CBHOs? How can these organizations and their advocacy efforts help eliminate health disparities? The two chapters in Part One begin to address those issues; Parts Two and Three further the discussion and provide some evidence to aid in responding to those questions.

Highlighted throughout both chapters is the critical function of forming partnerships to advocate for and deliver comprehensive, coordinated, and sustainable health care services amid changing social, political, cultural, and economic trends. These first chapters are intended to introduce and orient readers to the issues involved in providing health care from the perspective of the community, as a viable approach to health service delivery and to the theoretical anchors of that approach.

These chapters explain how community health needs have historically been met by organized advocacy efforts that emanate from both within and outside affected communities. As part of that explanation, Chapter One initiates a discussion on the need for CBHOs to build organizational capacity to advocate for improved health outcomes in their community that is further elaborated on in Chapter Five. An introductory discussion on how CBHOs work to develop, implement, and sustain programmatic and strategic responses to improve community health is also supplied in Chapter One but explored in depth in Chapters Four and Six, where information is also provided on how CBHOs handle the challenges inherent in attaining self-sufficiency. Finally, Chapters One and Two illustrate that as CBHOs engage in the various operations intended to eliminate existing health disparities, they must also contribute to communitywide development.

Historical and Organizational Frameworks of Community-Based Health Organizations in the United States

Marcia Bayne Smith

This chapter supplies working definitions of community-based health organizations (CBHOs) and their advocate role and then provides two frameworks, historical and organizational, that facilitate an examination of the role, purpose, and functions of CBHOs. Several concepts are introduced that increase our understanding of the many intangible attributes of health from the community perspective. These concepts—community organizing and the building of social capital, social cohesion, social glue, social bridges, the development of a strong civil society, and the community empowerment that follows—all play vital roles in the quality of life and the quality of health outcomes in any community. At the same time, these concepts point to specific areas of community development and empowerment in which CBHOs play a significant role.

Consequently, the chapter also looks at the historical development of community health, leading up to the emergence and growth of CBHOs. It also looks at the organization and structure of CBHOs and their capacity for empowering communities through development of partnerships that improve health outcomes and other community conditions.

Learning Objectives

- Social, economic, political, cultural, legal, and linguistic forces influence the shape and delivery of health services in general and the development of CBHOs in particular in a given community.
- The growth or demise of community health services is subject to competing national, regional, and local interests, as well as the historical journey unique to each community.
- A receptive political climate, strong social capital, social cohesion, a civil society, and a well-organized advocacy network are essential for community health services to advance.
- The development of community health services in the United States has undergone two major stages and is now entering a third.
- There is renewed interest in neighborhood-based health centers as effective service delivery models, particularly in urban settings, as a result of immigration and migration, the replacement of manufacturing jobs with service sector jobs, and restructured levels of federal and state support to cities.
- The role of government in the development of CBHOs continues to change.
- Improvement in community health outcomes requires that CBHOs develop the technological capacity to plan, advocate, deliver, monitor, and evaluate culturally acceptable preventive and primary services.

Working Definitions

It is important, before discussing important concepts, that all participants have a clear idea of precisely what those concepts mean. To that end, I provide here some definitions of the most important terms we will be encountering throughout this book.

Community-Based Health Organizations

Community-based health organizations are formal, legal structures established by, or together with, community residents, in order to advocate for, secure, increase access to, or provide health and health-related social support services to a community. There are two distinguishing characteristics of CBHOs. The first is their unique ability to serve as a bridge between their constituents and mainstream service delivery systems, thus facilitating access to care. The second is their ability to use their knowledge and cultural identity to build reciprocal relationships with a broad range of government health, social service, civic, educational, and religious institutions to foster coordinated, comprehensive, and culturally appropriate services.

The term *community-based health organizations* is intended to impart the basic philosophical precept of neighborhood-based or locally based entities providing health and social support services to communities or defined populations. CBHOs are presented here not as a category unto themselves but as a subset of *community-based organizations* (CBOs). The primary focus or mission of CBHOs is to intervene in eliminating the causes of poor health as opposed to focusing solely on the health problems themselves. In this context, they provide health education, outreach, and case management services, and sometimes they do so in conjunction with clinical care.

Community

Community is defined here as a group of people who share a geographical space; have common social bonds of status, concerns, or perspectives about specific issues; and assume, depending on the depth and strength of social capital available in that community, the obligations and responsibilities involved in collectively helping one another (Rubin and Rubin, 2001).

Community-Based

Community-based suggests a cadre of residents who, with the involvement of fellow residents, institutions, and other stakeholders, take on a central role in building and empowering their community and its organizations. The synergy that results from community-based involvement helps garner communitywide involvement and sustain collective efforts in public health actions around concerns identified by residents. *Community-based* is also indicative of collective activities of residents anchored within their community. For example, a hospital may be located in the community but would not be considered community-based because its support, stakeholders, staff, trustees, and investors may not necessarily come from that community.

Community Influence

How does the community influence health and health behaviors within it? From a sociological perspective, humans do not live in a disorganized fashion. Although we make individual and personal decisions all the time, we can do so only in the context of the family, community, city, country, and larger world in which we live. Sociology has taught us that our social world guides our behavior and life choices in much the same way that the seasons influence our clothing and activities (Macionis, 2005). Another answer, from an urban planning point of view, says, quite simply, that your health is influenced by where you live. It would appear, then, that regardless of the perspective, one's environment or community becomes critically important in terms of its ability to influence health behaviors, activities, and ultimately health outcomes.

Knowledge of how community influences health helps us in various ways. For one thing, it helps us think critically about various "truths." Many of the "truths" that abound about health are not necessarily factual. For example, a popular belief during the 1970s and 1980s was the notion that we are each individually and solely responsible for our own health. Because that idea was accepted by policymakers, it not only drove health policy but also made it easier to blame victims of certain illnesses and praise healthier people for their willpower or superior health behaviors (Byrd and Clayton, 1993). When we understand the influence of community on health, we are better able to think about our beliefs critically and to determine to what extent community or individual behaviors contribute to health outcomes and why.

Knowledge of how community influences health helps us determine how to work effectively within communities to address health concerns. Developing a deeper understanding of how community influences health can shed light on the various factors contributing to the disproportionate incidence of illness and disease among certain racial, ethnic, and socioeconomic groups and explain differences in the availability of funding and providers from one community to the next. As we understand more about the significant influence of community on health, we gain greater clarity in assessing health conditions in a given community. Often this newfound clarity leads to active involvement in development and pursuit of goals that will improve the health of a community.

Knowing how community influences health also helps us value the cultural diversity of every community. The rich diversity of the United States is the result of four centuries of immigration from around the world. There have always been ethnic enclaves of recent newcomers and distinct neighborhoods inhabited by descendants of previous immigrants. The residential pattern of ethnic enclaves helps community members maintain their cultural practices while functioning within the larger social milieu. As the size of an immigrant group grows, it eventually comes to include individuals identified as natural healers in whom the group places its trust regarding matters of health. In such communities, Western "biomedicine" is not necessarily the first course of action but frequently the treatment of last resort. One of the many lessons to be learned from cultural diversity is that group values and experiences influence health behaviors that affect health outcomes.

Health

In the preamble to its constitution, the World Health Organization defines *health* as "a state of complete physical, mental, and social well-being and not merely as the absence of disease or infirmity." This broad definition suggests that the well-being of any group of people cannot be viewed in isolation from its history and current conditions. However, the unwillingness to broaden the definition beyond a focus on disease and infirmity, and the repercussions for human health, is rooted in a dramatic shift in the way people viewed the world during the Age of Enlightenment, in the sixteenth and seventeenth centuries. That view, based on a method of "scientific" reasoning that is mechanistic and linear, is often referred to as Cartesian thinking or Cartesian reductionism (Cottingham, 1998; Payer, 1988). The Cartesian paradigm has exerted undue influence on shaping views in every sphere of life for some four hundred years. It is credited with development of the Western biomedical model that reduced health to mechanical functioning and established strict divisions between mind and body (Capra, 1982).

An important outgrowth of Cartesian reductionism is the contemporary biomedical model, which is essentially concerned with only four things: the diagnosis, the disease, the patient, and the treatment (Foss and Rothenberg, 1987), in that order. The biomedical model is ill-suited to addressing current community health needs in an advanced industrialized society like the United States, for two reasons. One has to do with new knowledge about the etiology of disease, which stresses that in addition to the early biological programming, chronic health risks result over the life course from adverse environments, childhood and adolescent illnesses, nutritional practices, levels of physical activity, and many other influences (Brunner, 2000). The other has to do with the fact that over the course of the past hundred years, infectious epidemics and pandemics have become less prevalent, replaced by chronic illnesses and new epidemics that are more closely associated with behaviors governed by social norms, habits, beliefs, and shared characteristics and perspectives.

As a result, despite the phenomenal scientific advancements and accomplishments in medicine in recent decades, the biomedical model has proved inadequate to address health-related behaviors and their health outcomes. The poor fit of this model with current health problems is particularly noticeable in non-Western and nonmainstream communities in the United States (Bayne Smith, 1996b). In fact, the biomedical definition of health as the absence of disease tended to ignore group history and in so doing did not address the idea of community health. As a result, it is only in the past twenty to thirty years that medicine in the United States has become concerned with the disparity in health between groups or communities or with the differences in population and community characteristics that can either contribute to or detract from improving health outcomes. As efforts are made to define health in more comprehensive terms, it is expected that the health of communities will be addressed.

Organization

An *organization* is an entity built by members of a community to gather and focus information, pressure government and private agencies, conduct protests, contribute to the empowerment of its members, or create new forms of ownership (Rubin and Rubin, 2001). Organizations bring resources and capacity to educate, empower, and mobilize a community and foster the development of CBHOs as organized, structured responses to health concerns.

Building organizations presents a difficult challenge for communities where civil society is weak, recollection of historic experiences is an obstacle, or resources, skills, and capacity are lacking. As a result, some communities must first focus on providing their constituents with social support services to assist them in breaking down barriers that stand in the way of their quest for a community organization to provide health services.

Health Advocate

A *health advocate* seeks to influence decisions about health policy and the allocation of health resources in order to improve community health outcomes. As health advocates, CBHOs employ organized strategies and actions while holding themselves accountable to the communities on whose behalf they advocate.

Health advocates strive to improve health outcomes for their community by gaining a voice and a place at the table of relevant institutions and agencies where decisions affecting community health are made. The strength of CBHO advocacy efforts lies in the fact that access issues are felt most acutely at the local level. Therefore, CBHOs are in a unique position to articulate social issues that affect health as well as local approaches to health improvement. In this context, their goal is to change the relationships of power between centers of decision making and the people and communities affected by those decisions.

Since the terrorist attacks of September 11, 2001, perceptions of health and the impact of political, social, and economic events on the health of a given community have changed. As a result, along with new concerns about air pollution and air quality and the availability, supply, and quality of vaccines against smallpox, anthrax, and various other biological and chemical agents, there are also new concerns about "community health." In that regard, the very presence of nuclear power plants in our communities seems now more than ever to pose an increased health threat. In this environment of heightened awareness of terrorism, one of the equally pressing health needs that has surfaced is for ongoing mental health services at a time when resources for mental health services in several states and communities have either been reduced or evaporated entirely. Though sometimes considered not as tangible as physical health, the mental health and other nonphysical characteristics of communities carry important ramifications for the health of a community.

Community Health

Before we can define *community health,* we must recognize that in the United States, some communities are subject to greater environmental health risks and deficits, such as low social capital and weak civil society, as a result of distinct population characteristics. The residents of these communities are not only assigned a lower rank in the U.S. social hierarchy but are also at greater distance politically and economically from all those above them. In addition, residents of these communities tend not to form advocacy organizations, nor are they part of social networks that can facilitate access to services and resources relative to their health care needs (Murray, Frenk, and Gakidou, 2001). It is in these communities that CBHOs are well positioned to organize residents and focus their efforts. The emphasis must be on the building of social capital and social cohesion and on community development and empowerment resulting from an engaged civil society. The desired end product is empowered communities that develop the organizational capacity to advocate for improved health outcomes.

Community Building, Social Capital, Social Cohesion, and Civil Society

The term *community building* broadly describes the work of organizing a community and creating linkages at various levels. The concept of building *social capital* is more complex. Social capital is not the same as economic capital. Economic capital is most often measured individually, whereas social capital is a collective assessment of specific kinds of resources within a community, group, or society. Thus *capital* in a community context refers to the supply of less discernible resources: trust, duty, reciprocity, responsibility, obligation, and control. In the absence of these intangible forms of social capital, communities, groups, and sometimes whole societies become disorganized and destabilized.

Similarly, *social cohesion* is a collective or ecological measure of a community. Ichiro Kawachi and Lisa Berkman (2000) explain that social cohesion refers to the absence of latent group conflict and the presence of strong social bonds (capital) and a strong civil society. *Civil society* is used to describe the web of voluntary groups and associations that exist in empowered, well-developed communities. Civil society serves as a bridge between people and government to protect people, help meet needs unmet by government, and function as the social glue that holds society together (Kawachi and Berkman, 2000). The significance of these terms lies in their connection to health outcomes, demonstrated through a body of research that has emerged over the past four decades (Schoenbach, Kaplan, Fredman, and Kleinbaum, 1986; Wilkinson, 1996; and Kawachi and others, 1996). Research to determine how social capital, social cohesion, and civil society help build community and move it toward the goal of improving health outcomes must include studies that examine poor health outcomes in communities with diminished social capital (Berkman and Syme, 1979), communities in which social capital and social cohesion exert a positive influence on the use of preventive health services (Kawachi and Berkman, 2000), and organized advocacy efforts in socially cohesive communities that have been shown to preserve community programs and services intended to be derailed by budget cuts (Coleman, 1988).

Given these explanations of community-related concepts, how is health defined from a community perspective? To do this, it is necessary to consider the larger milieu in which a given community is embedded, including economic development, quality of education, religion, hopes, goals, government structures, and cultural customs. It is equally important to weigh some of the emerging and controversial areas, such as the association between health outcomes and the social capital, social cohesion, and civil society in a given community.

Consequently, the definition of community health goes beyond the "absence of disease" paradigm to place greater emphasis on the "whole person within the environment" configuration. This broader, more encompassing definition, in which health is seen as connected to community, has long been understood by many health advocates as having direct import for the kinds of approaches used to deliver services. The broader definitions of community health have been the basis of arguments used by proponents since the 1940s to advance the idea of moving the nation toward health service delivery models known as community-oriented primary care or community medicine (Kark and Abramson, 1982).

Community Health, CBHOs, and Advocacy

Most community residents and some of the health professionals that serve them are very aware that community health is affected by a host of factors. Some of these factors include culture, traditions, the status of women, rates of unemployment, and domestic violence; levels of hopelessness, social cohesion, and social capital; the strength of civil society; increasing rates of sexually transmitted diseases, including HIV/AIDS; and environmental injustice (Bayne Smith, 1996b; Kawachi and Berkman, 2000; Putnam, 1993; Gamble, 2002; Freudenberg, 1984).

Residents living in low-income, racial, ethnic, immigrant, and other underserved communities have been organizing for half a century to create CBHOs to address their own long-standing health problems. The challenge is how to structure mutually beneficial arrangements among community residents, health professionals both in and outside of government, and the health industry as a whole, in an effort to deliver a range of primary care and social support services to many different types of communities.

Unlike community residents and their CBHOs, health agencies and departments at city, state, or federal levels have only recently recognized the wide-ranging factors affecting community health. Although the process of recognition has been slow, the fact that there is movement toward incorporating community into the definition and programming of health services is encouraging. As government health systems pay more attention to community health services, their efforts are fueled by an emerging body of research that carefully documents the important connections between the health and economic status of a community, its access to health care, and associations between aspects of work and health (Leon and Walt, 2001; Engels, [1845] 1987; Marmot and others, 1997;

Bayne Smith, Graham, Mason, and Drossman, 2004; Bayne Smith and others, 2004; Leigh, Jimenez, Lee, and Andrews, 2002). Much of the movement that we currently witness on the part of government health systems is due in large measure to increased community advocacy to secure health services. Of critical significance to the advocacy efforts on the part of communities is the interpretation of the word *organization* and its importance to the term *CBHO*.

Questions About CBHOs and Advocacy

Why study CBHOs? The most significant reason for studying CBHOs is simply that CBHOs represent a key component of successful health delivery in the United States. Surprisingly, there is a dearth of literature on the subject. Unquestionably, much has been written about different kinds of community-based services, including primary and ambulatory care, emergency care, complementary and alternative medical care, and home health care. There is also an abundant literature on community health centers (CHCs). However, CBHOs are a distinct model of community-based health services that places critical emphasis on resident involvement in defining not only community health needs but also the responses generated.

Faced with long-term, persistent challenges in addressing health disparities, U.S. health providers and policymakers are reluctantly and slowly being forced to see that to serve culturally diverse populations more effectively, greater emphasis must be placed on a community-oriented vision of primary care, rather than on hospital-based care. As a result, after investing heavily for almost a century in the development of hospital-based services, the health care industry has been forced in the past twenty-five years to move away from caring for patients in the hospital setting and provide more services in the ambulatory care setting. These changes continue to be driven by a combination of recent demographic trends in the United States and market forces such as managed care organizations (MCOs).

Understanding that the shift to community-based care has not been uniform across the U.S. population led us to inquire about the importance of advocacy as an important function of CBHOs. Statistics on health care utilization from the National Center for Health Statistics (NCHS) at the Centers for Disease Control and

Prevention (CDC) (2003, tab. 83; McCaig and Ly, 2002) were useful in shedding some light on the importance of advocacy:

- The rates of visits to physicians differ by age, gender, race, socioeconomic status, and insurance.
- In 1998, Americans age seventy-five and older had the highest number of ambulatory care visits, 764 visits per 100 persons.
- Women made 1.4 visits to a physician for every visit by a man.
- Whites had more visits to physicians' offices than blacks.
- More blacks than whites used the emergency room or a hospital outpatient department as their primary source of care in 2000, indicating a lack of both insurance coverage and a regular source of care.

Although mandatory Medicaid managed care did increase physician visits for the poor, one of its intended goals was to decrease emergency room visits, and it has not done so. Further, the population of the United States grew by 3.8 percent over the past decade, but the number of emergency room visits increased from 90.5 million in 1994 to 94.8 million in 1998, representing a 4.75 percent increase in just four years (Mezey, 2002, p. 185). Moreover, while approximately 47 percent of the patients receiving emergency care in 2000 had an urgent or emergent condition, the other half did not need the expensive, intense resources of an emergency room (McCaig and Ly, 2002).

The advocacy work of CBHOs on behalf of underserved communities is in part aimed at rectifying these statistics. CBHOs have traditionally advocated for the uninsured to balance market forces driving the managed care (MC) and Medicaid managed care (MMC) organizations that do not extend insurance coverage to everyone. The uninsured are the group for which there is greatest concern, and they are one of the groups that are most often served by CBHOs. In addition to the serious problems of access to care for the uninsured and the heavy reliance on and inappropriate use of emergency rooms that continues, there is a deeper concern regarding the cultural and linguistic appropriateness of managed care services at the community level. CBHOs provide an alternative, as they are largely representative of the communities they serve.

The advocacy efforts of CBHOs becomes even more significant in view of the fact that to date, MC and MMC organizations have not established a notable record of accomplishment in reaching out and involving community leaders in policy and decision-making capacities. This is something that CBHOs have been successful at doing. Because of their success, CBHOs have also reached out to explore and develop partnerships with managed care organizations that can ultimately expand the reach of MC and MMC organizations into communities they did not historically serve, while at the same time enhancing the capacity of CBHOs. This trend is expected to continue and requires careful study.

Although it must be acknowledged that some positive movement is occurring, serious concerns remain. A recent report of the Institute of Medicine (2003) of the National Academies indicates that racial and ethnic minorities tend to receive a lower quality of health care than nonminorities, even when controlling for access factors such as health insurance and income, and that the sources of these disparities are rooted in the complexity of past and current inequities involving the entire health system bureaucracy, from administrators to all levels of health care professionals, as well as the patients themselves.

In the face of unrelenting health disparities in the United States, what can CBHOs in their role as health advocates do to help eliminate them? To answer this question, we employ two different frameworks. The first examines historical developments in community-based health services, primarily in the United States, and discusses some of the initial concepts, policies, and programs on which CBHOs now rest. The second framework looks at how CBHOs are organized and examines their roles and functions particularly as they relate to resource requirements, consumer needs, and types of service provided.

Historical Framework: Development of Community Health Services in the United States

Evidence exists that from the very earliest civilizations, humans have been concerned with community health. As early as 25,000 B.C., carvings showing physical deformities were made on cave walls in Spain. Later Chinese carvings on tortoise shells depict health practices in the Xia and Shang dynasties (twenty-first to eleventh centuries B.C.) and also the digging of water wells and ditches (Green and Ottoson, 1994). Excavated sites of communities thousands of years old have revealed bathrooms, drains, covered sewers, and drinking water supply systems in societies of the Nile region, in ancient Indian cities, and throughout the Greco-Roman world (Green and Ottoson, 1994; Rosen, 1958).

Lessons from the Past

One of the great lessons regarding community health dates from the Late Middle Ages. In 1095, the Christian Byzantine emperor Alexius I asked Pope Urban II for help in expelling the Muslim Seljuk Turks, who were invading his empire (in Asia Minor, modern Turkey) from the east. The pope willingly complied and decided that if his Christian armies were going that far, they might as well continue on to Jerusalem and "liberate" the Christian holy places there, thus initiating nearly two centuries of religious wars between Christianity and Islam known as the Crusades (Spielvogel, 2005). The massive movement of troops and other people from one region to another during the Crusades contributed to large-scale health problems. Diseases such as cholera, bubonic plague, and pulmonary anthrax spread from one country to another along the migrants' path, killing thousands of people. In addition, as trade routes opened up and ships moved from one port to another in Asia, Africa, Europe, and the Middle East, infectious diseases traveled with them. Drastic measures had to be taken at the time to prevent epidemics. Some European nations instituted quarantine stations and ordered newcomers to remain there for several months until they were deemed free of disease. These measures were not highly effective (McNeill, 1977).

The sixteenth century ushered in the Enlightenment (1600–1800), and with it came an initial understanding of disease processes. Although the twentieth century brought relief from the earlier pandemics and epidemics, it ended with the emergence of new epidemics (HIV/AIDS) and potential epidemics (Ebola, SARS). Note that throughout history, most pandemics and epidemics have been interpreted as divine punishment for the sins of humans. Nevertheless, we have abundant evidence of carefully planned, if misguided, public health efforts aimed at protecting the community, even during the Dark Ages. It appears, then, that there has been some level of recognition for millennia that although there was some individual responsibility for health, there was also the need for some societal or communitywide approach. In fact, most of the earliest public health activity was born out of the recognition that when faced with transmissible diseases, preventive action at the community level is necessary.

The U.S. Context

From 1600 to the mid-1800s, major European countries set out to colonize the rest of the world, including what is now the United States. Colonization had an impact on the health of every new group encountered as populations around the world were introduced to theretofore unknown diseases. Sometimes infectious disease like measles was even spread intentionally to aid in the subjugation of a population, as was the case when the Spanish colonized South America. Later, once the new order had been established, the European nation might provide whatever remedies were in fashion. Similar stories were played out on the African continent.

The taking of the North American continent was facilitated to a large extent by that familiar process. As a result of European diseases, the Huron nation was reduced by half, 90 percent of the native population along the East Coast were killed, and the Eskimo and Inuit populations of the Alaskan regions were seriously reduced (Green and Ottoson, 1994). The fact that there was a concerted U.S. military strategy to decimate and subdue survivors of the Native American population and appropriate their land cannot be denied. However, health conditions undoubtedly contributed to the fact that by 1836, many of the remaining tribes readily signed treaties with the U.S. government in which they relinquished millions of acres of land in exchange for medical supplies, physician services, and promises of hospital construction (Kaufman and Joseph-Fox, 1996). In summary, disease eliminated much of the opposition to the early colonizers and later facilitated the European conquest of the American continents with much less bloodshed than had been anticipated.

People in the United States during the colonial era and the early days of the republic also suffered from pandemics of such diseases as yellow fever, smallpox, measles, typhus, and scarlet fever that resulted in deaths in the tens of thousands. These outbreaks ended only after they had run their course through a given population or locale. Some colonies took action by setting up citizens' committees to provide communitywide direction for responding to a pandemic, but this kind of guidance was usually ineffective. For the most part, there was little capacity or effort in the colonial years to develop health policy on any uniform or consistent scale. Individual colonies took small steps to require the mandatory recording of births and deaths, but this was a time when life expectancy rarely exceeded forty-five years, health science and health services were unheard of, and community action regarding health occurred only as a response to outbreaks.

Health care in colonial communities, such as it was, occurred essentially through local efforts of residents to address the health concerns and events they faced, as no government health systems existed. Nevertheless, throughout the colonies, in almost every culture or group, health events such as births were treated as community events. Slave women gave birth to their children assisted by midwives who were themselves slaves. In fact, the midwifery skills of these slave women were relied on by both black and white women (Holmes, 1986). For some Native American women, childbirth was also a community event in which they were assisted by their mothers, mothers-in-law, and midwives (Axtell, 1981).

The spread of infectious disease due to the overcrowded and unsanitary living and working conditions of the Industrial Revolution led to both Engel's radical analysis of the condition of the working classes in Manchester, England ([1845] 1987), and Chadwick's more liberal analysis and report on the health of British workers ([1842] 1965). Engel's analysis blamed the deterioration of health on the rise of capitalism, whereas Chadwick suggested that the deterioration was due to poor sanitation. Chadwick's analysis resulted in the development of boards of health in London, Manchester, and Liverpool in England between 1825 and 1846 and later to boards of health in Massachusetts and New York. A similar examination of the health situation in the northeastern United States by Shattuck (1848) in the mid-nineteenth century served as a guide for the development of public health services in every town and city up through the state level. Ongoing scientific developments, particularly in bacteriology, also forced significant changes in approaches to public health. One of the most significant changes was that medicine gained a larger measure of control and prevention over infectious diseases.

New Challenges for Public Health

By the third decade of the twentieth century, it became clear that there was a need to begin shifting health resources and other health investments away from infectious diseases, not only into the arenas of personal and individual health but also into community and public health. This would include health promotion and disease prevention services to achieve a balance with the scientific and technological advancements that were well under way. The shift did not occur, and the balance was never struck due largely to the medical profession's continuing efforts from the mid-nineteenth to mid-twentieth centuries to consolidate its authority and become a powerful political force (Starr, 1982). The increasing power of organized medicine resulted in a growth of resources for the development of hospitals, the training of physicians and other health personnel, and biomedical research.

Some analysts believe that as the medical profession became more powerful, public health services suffered. Garrett (2000) contends that during the first two decades of the twentieth century, public health began a downward spiral because of two historical events. One was the implementing of polio quarantines in New York City when only a vaccine would eventually prevent the disease. The other was physicians' countering of Prohibition by readily prescribing alternatives such as opium, laudanum, belladonna, absinthe, marijuana, and cocaine. In defense of public health, it must be noted that although all societies suffer ups and downs in public health, the United States was successful in conquering polio and many other diseases.

As a result of the growth and consolidation process in the medical profession, public health was forced to shift its focus from larger environmental and social issues to personal hygiene and the transmission of infectious diseases, which required more reliance on the techniques of medicine. A main source of the territorial conflict between medicine and public health in the early decades of the twentieth century was the reluctance of doctors in private practice to meet reporting requirements for infectious diseases, such as tuberculosis and venereal disease. In addition, many doctors in private practice, supported by fees for service, did not see the need to cooperate with public health authorities in the establishment of publicly supported health centers for coordinating preventive medical treatment for individuals who could not afford to pay a private fee (Starr, 1982).

Thus it was clear by the early twentieth century that the poor were increasingly marginalized and did not benefit equitably from advancements in health care because initially the major source of care for the poor was charity, followed gradually by local government responsibility for indigent care (Williams and Torrens, 1999). Public health nurses and voluntary health agencies historically provided outreach, education, and some primary care services in poor communities, but by the 1930s, there were huge differences in health status, based on class, race, and ethnicity, as well as between urban and rural communities (La Viest, 2002). It had also become clear that changes in U.S. immigration policies in the 1960s led to changes in the demographic makeup of the nation, creating dense concentrations of nonwhite native-born and immigrant populations, especially in its larger urban metropolises. These multiple population segments of racial and ethnic groups, immigrants, and the poor and near-poor contribute to the difficulty of gaining access to the many benefits of Western medicine in a culturally acceptable service delivery format.

Community Health in a Diverse Nation

Initial efforts to deal with the growing disparity in health suffered by the poor tended to be made by concerned community members. Government support and programs would follow, but much later. The development of public health services in New York City provides a clear and typical example of this trend in the delivery of health services to new immigrant populations.

Throughout the nineteenth century, the New York City Council would establish a board of health during an outbreak of disease; once the disease had subsided, the board would be allowed to disappear. Volunteer reformers, made up mostly of middle- and upper-class New Yorkers, advocated for and were able to garner the required political support to eventually establish a permanent department of health in the city. A major catalyst for these advocacy efforts was the deplorable housing conditions of the ever-increasing numbers of immigrants in the city. Reformers focused the city's attention on the growing problems of slum housing, in which the population was increasing by an average of 250,000 immigrants per year between 1866 and 1870 (Duffy, 1974, p. 191).

Health problems associated with infectious diseases such as yellow fever, cholera, tuberculosis, and smallpox continued during the remaining years of the nineteenth century. Each shipload of immigrants that pulled into a New York City port therefore delivered a potential health hazard. Early efforts by New York City to quarantine new arrivals were later taken over by state quarantine officers, who improved processing and screening standards by the beginning of the twentieth century, making it possible to provide health services to new arrivals with infectious diseases (Duffy, 1974, p. 199).

A century later, New York City again became a city overflowing with new immigrants. The Hart-Cellar Immigration Act of 1965 superseded the quota system of the McCarran-Walter Act of 1924 and for the first time in U.S. history dramatically increased the numbers of immigrants from non-Indo-European countries, albeit temporarily. In 1985, immigration reform changed the laws once again to restrict the flow of nonwhite immigrants. Even so, as of 1995, an estimated 33 percent of the city's population was foreign-born, and approximately another 20 percent were the offspring of immigrants (New York City Department of City Planning, 1996, p. 14). Health services to immigrants now had a completely different focus. The newest immigrants and the New York City ethnic immigrant enclaves into which they moved faced a radically different set of health issues than their counterparts did a century earlier. Health problems for the most recent newcomers, as for the general population, consisted primarily of long-term chronic diseases rather than short-term infectious diseases. At the same time, the new arrivals also faced complicated new immigration laws that served to limit and even block their access to health care services.

By the 1960s, the nation had eradicated most of the worst infectious diseases in the United States, and in 1977, the global community experienced its last case of smallpox (Hopkins, 1989). Looking back, we now realize that recognition of this success by the medical community in the late 1970s contributed to drastic reductions in budgets for health promotion and education. Unfortunately, this occurred immediately prior to the onslaught of the HIV/AIDS pandemic of the early 1980s. Moreover, these budget cuts, together with restrictions on immigrant health care entitlement benefits, served to discourage the use of preventive services by the poor, newly arrived, and underserved.

Unmet Health Needs

With or without government resources, communities have always devised methods to deal with illness. For example, Native Americans had abundant healing practices, focused on balancing the physical, spiritual, emotional, and social aspects of the individual. Sickness was seen as an imbalance, an absence of harmony (Kaufman and Joseph-Fox, 1996). These beliefs were at odds with mainstream American medicine, whose views were voiced by Dr. Benjamin Rush in a paper titled "An Inquiry into the Natural History of Medicine Among the Indians," written in 1793, in which he concluded that "we have no discoveries in the *materia medica* to hope for from the Indians in North-America." Despite disparaging criticisms from learned men, "Indian cures" were quite popular and marketable among the general public.

As we now know, much greater by comparison than the decimation of Native American tribes through warfare and the submersion of Indian culture was the neglect of their health needs. In fact, the spread of tuberculosis, trachoma, and other diseases among the Native peoples eventually prompted such public outrage that President Taft urged Congress in 1921 to pass the Snyder Act, mandating congressional appropriations for the "relief of distress and conservation of health" among Native Americans (Kaufman and Joseph-Fox, 1996).

Unmet Health Needs and Mainstream Medicine:
Two Major Concerns

A long-standing concern in the health arena has to do with the economic controls exercised by the health care industry. Health service delivery in the United States was ad hoc and uncoordinated until the beginning of the twentieth century. However, even before there was any significant level of professional organization among practitioners of medicine, they viewed the poor as useful in terms of training and practice opportunities but evinced little desire to provide ongoing medical care for them, due primarily to financial considerations. This unwillingness to serve the poor deepened over time and became so strong that between 1870 and 1910, the poorer states lost physicians relative to population while the wealthier states gained them. For example, in 1870, there was one doctor for every 894 residents in South Carolina, compared to one doctor for every 712 residents in Massachusetts; by 1910, the number of residents per doctor had risen to 1,170 in South Carolina and fallen to 497 in Massachusetts (Starr, 1982, pp. 124–125).

The second concern regarding unmet health needs and mainstream medicine follows the first, because economics and politics are inextricably intertwined. The ability of organized medicine to protect its economic interests flows in no small measure from its reinvention as an organized political entity. The health care industry became organized politically by the mid-1960s, with sufficient lobbying power to influence legislation to protect its interests. However, this very ability on the part of organized medicine begs the question of the distribution of political power in a so-called democracy. The concern here, notwithstanding the intent of organized medicine to protect its interests, is that the unmet health needs of certain groups and communities in the United States appear to be directly proportionate to the level of political power those groups exercise in the society. In a study on political empowerment and health status of African Americans conducted in 176 cities in thirty-two states, Thomas La Viest (1992) measured black political power in two ways: relative black political power, which is the proportion of blacks on the city council divided by the proportion of blacks in the voting-age population, and absolute black political power, which is the percentage of city council members who are black, indicating the level at which African Americans are empowered to control the political and policymaking apparatus of the city. The study confirmed the hypothesis that a higher level of black political power relative to the black voting-age population is associated with lower black postneonatal mortality, but absolute black political power is not (see also Dye and Renick, 1981).

Understanding Why Health Needs Go Unmet

The historical lack of political will or interest on the part of decision makers in addressing the health needs of the poor, newcomers, and the uninsured and underinsured has not changed in almost a century. Why? Several reasons stand out, the first of which is that poverty makes excessive demands on the poor for their day-to-day survival leaving them with few material resources and little physical energy to invest in advocacy and political activity, which are the only ways to effect political change. Second, a large number of newcomers reside in poor communities, and lacking U.S. citizenship upon arrival, they are unable to influence the political process through the power of their vote. This is to say they have no political power through which to lobby for social change for at least the first five years they legally reside in the United States. The third reason encompasses the first two in that the combined forces of poverty, noncitizenship, and a lack of acculturation render some poor communities marginalized and uninitiated politically, and so they are not always aware that health care must be regarded as a human right and a public good. Neither do they understand that the means by which human rights and public goods are distributed is political, requiring political participation and the acquisition of advocacy skills.

Far worse than the slow development of organized political approaches to issues affecting their community are the attitudes toward elections and politics held by many members of the voting public. Their diminishing presence at the polls over the past few decades reflects feelings of apathy, bitterness, distrust, and disenchantment with the political process and the empty promises of elected officials. These sentiments are evident in all sectors of the population, regardless of income, race, gender, or locality, but it is most counterproductive for the poor, who have the least access to services and other resources and public goods in U.S. society. In addition, elected officials feel free to ignore poor communities because of the perception that they don't vote.

Another compelling reason that the health needs of some communities remain unmet is that the most recent newcomer groups differ greatly in terms of race, language, ethnicity, and culture, from the German, Irish, Jewish, and Italian immigrant groups who came in the late 1800s and early 1900s. Most of these immigrants were fair-skinned Europeans, not too different from the majority populations already settled in the United States. They could blend in fairly easily. This is not true for many of the more recent newcomers. Being nonwhite has always constituted a major marker of difference in the United States.

Historically, race in the United States has served as the basis for denial of social justice and access to resources and critical services. However, it is now of serious concern that in the opening decade of the twenty-first century, the burden of health disparities in the nation continues to fall primarily on the poor, a disproportionate number of whom are members of racial and ethnic populations. The significance of this difference and its impact on access to care becomes even more pronounced in view of the fact that in 1965, when immigration opened up to permit entry of racially and ethnically different newcomers, the majority of health policymakers, physicians, and industry leaders in the 1960s and 1970s were predominantly white and male. These health leaders, for the most part, have historically been the least knowledgeable about how to serve people who are culturally, racially, or ethnically different.

In addition, poor people lack the resources necessary to practice preventive health care. In the case of immigrants, they also lack knowledge about the complexity of the U.S. health care system and hence feel intimidated by it. The result is a deep-seated reluctance to make use of the U.S. health care system except in emergencies. Another source of reluctance to use mainstream health services is the presence among some racial and ethnic groups of their own healers and practitioners of culturally based health customs, such as Santeria, Candomble, and Voodoo (Gregory, 1987). Further, the relative ease of travel today facilitates access to all of the culturally prescribed tools, equipment, and other resources required to maintain customary health practices, beneficial or not (Korin, 1985).

Community Responses

Whether the issue is barriers to health care access or cultural preferences in terms of health care practices and behaviors, several studies have documented the disproportionately worse health status among the poor, underserved, immigrant, and uninsured populations in both urban and rural settings (Fruchter, Boyce, and Hunt, 1980; O'Toole, Gibbon, Hanusa, and Fine, 1999; see also Fruchter and others, 1980). Activists, advocates, and organizers in poor communities across the United States had become increasingly aware by the late 1960s of the negative health conditions in their neighborhoods.

In response to this situation, many of these communities did what other marginalized groups have done historically in the absence of family ties, supportive relationships, or the assistance of the larger society: they developed their own community-based organizations to address their unmet health needs. And these community-based organizations became the harbingers of CBHOs. In some poor communities, CBHOs continue to serve as the primary resource for health, social support, and immigration-related services (Bayne Smith, 1996a).

Developing local mechanisms to meet community needs is not a new response. In the twentieth century, working-class immigrants on Manhattan's Lower East Side contracted with five hundred physicians to provide medical services to members of their organizations and benevolent societies (Sardell, 1988). The Cincinnati Social Unit Plan was developed toward the end of the Progressive Era (around 1918) by activists and residents in poor areas to provide a variety of services including health services. The small-scale success of this program aroused opposition from doctors, however, and the Cincinnati Plan soon faded away (Betten and Austin, 1990). Other underserved groups also developed local community-based efforts to respond to health needs. The National Medical Association (NMA), an organization of black physicians, and the Medical Committee for Human Rights (MCHR), organized by both black and white health professionals to provide medical services in various southern states during the civil rights era, coordinated health projects with local black and medical community workers. By 1966, the MCHR had branches in thirty northern and southern cities (McBride, 1994). Despite an ongoing struggle to build capacity and to acquire sufficient resources, local CBHOs continue to be a primary source of health care in their communities.

Government Support of Community Health Services: Two Phases of Development

Throughout U.S. history, communities have designed a variety of ways to respond to the health care needs of its residents. Those responses evolved into different structures, depending on the needs of the community being served; the skills, resources, and commitment they are able to garner from community stakeholders; and the social, political, and economic climate at the time those responses were being developed. As noted earlier, for most poor communities, the usual pattern of accessing health care was first to develop a local community-based health service and eventually, with the input and support of concerned members of the middle and upper classes, exert political pressure to ultimately obtain government support.

The push for government support went through two broad phases. In the lengthy first phase, political advocacy and activism helped establish some responses to local health needs of the poor in the eighteenth and nineteenth centuries. These responses occurred primarily in the form of dispensaries and the development of outpatient departments in hospitals. It must be noted, however, that by the time dispensaries met their demise in the early 1900s, local departments of health in large cities such as New York were already experimenting with the establishment of health district centers to provide medical care to residents, especially maternal and children's health care. Here too, as was done with dispensaries, organized medicine moved quickly to limit not only public funding for health district centers but also the kinds of health services that could be offered. The combined forces of these two actions served to drastically cut back the operations of most health district centers by the mid-1950s (Sardell, 1988).

In the second phase, advocates of community health services persevered in developing policy networks. Their efforts eventually gained congressional mandates allowing several forms of community health services to resurface by 1965 and again in the 1970s, each time with a different configuration, name, and government classification.

Phase 1: Dispensaries and Maternal Child Health Programs

The first phase of government support for health care services at the community level was influenced heavily by events in eighteenth-century England, where the first dispensary, known as the Dispensary of the Infant Poor, opened in London in 1769 (Rosen, 1958). The dispensary model was later transferred to the United States and became the major source of free and subsequently low-cost medical care and medications for the poor. Prior to the arrival of dispensaries in the United States, health care delivered by physicians was provided in the homes of wealthy patients who could afford to pay doctors to make house calls (Ehrenreich and English, 1973). However, dispensaries proved to be acceptable in meeting the health care needs of the poor and did so from the latter part of the eighteenth century through the first few decades of the twentieth century (Sardell, 1988). At the same time that health care was being provided for the poor in dispensaries, health services for the rich—and indeed the entire health care delivery system—was moving from the home to hospitals. The oldest hospitals were initially developed as alms houses to serve the poor (Rosner, 1979). These include Pennsylvania Hospital in Philadelphia, built in 1751; New York Hospital in New York City, built in 1791; and general hospitals in Baltimore, Cincinnati, and Savannah built in 1825 (Rosen, 1958).

By the early decades of the twentieth century, the convergence of increased scientific knowledge, discoveries of new medicines and treatment capabilities, and improved surgical methods all became centralized. Health care personnel were brought together with the rapidly emerging technologies in one place: hospitals. This concentration of resources ushered in the role of hospitals as the hub of all health-related activity in the nation (Williams and Torrens, 1999). Unfortunately, as hospitals blossomed into this new role, by the 1920s, dispensaries disappeared.

Alice Sardell (1988) suggests two major reasons for the demise of dispensaries. One can be found in the way they were structured. Dispensaries functioned as outpatient clinics serving as a training site for young physicians. When the Flexner Report on medical education in the United States and Canada was published in 1910, it forced major changes in the teaching of medicine following the European model, creating a focus on the sciences and research that was best anchored in modern hospitals. The other reason dispensaries did not survive is that the newly created and energized medical societies organized politically to conduct a campaign, beginning in 1890, against "dispensary abuse" by individuals who could afford to pay for care. The fundamental goal, of course, was to do away with any competition, as the majority of U.S. physicians were already practicing fee-for-service medicine, outside of hospitals, by the last part of the nineteenth century. The political campaign against dispensaries resulted in a 1899 law mandating that poor families undergo means testing to determine their eligibility for dispensary services.

This law created, in effect, a "two-class" system of health services (Sardell, 1988). Means testing went on to become firmly entrenched in the United States as the preferred method for rationing health or any other form of benefits or services for the poor.

In addition to dispensaries, early maternal child health (MCH) programs were significant. As early as 1912, the Children's Bureau, a federal agency, was established out of concerns about child labor and child abuse. As a result of the work of that agency, particularly its reports on the high incidence of maternal and infant mortality, legislation in the 1920s and 1930s authorized grants to the states to provide medical services to mothers and children; these services were usually provided at local health district centers. Later, the Social Security Act of 1935 established federal-state cooperative programs to provide preventive health services in the areas of MCH, crippled children, and child welfare (Davis and Millman, 1983). MCH programs, designed to reduce maternal and infant mortality, were substantially altered over the course of the next forty years through amendments that added a variety of other health categories. From its inception, MCH programs and the many other services provided under the MCH umbrella have been a source of struggle between state and local health agencies.

Phase 2: Federally Funded Community Health Programs

The second critical phase of government support for community-based health services occurred in two stages: from the mid-1960s to the mid-1970s and from the mid-1970s to the present. The first stage grew out of the Johnson administration's War on Poverty. The Economic Opportunity Act of 1964 established the Office of Economic Opportunity (OEO), and radically new policies were put in place to implement the Neighborhood Health Center program and later the Community Health Center program that would make health care and other services available to the poor.

The Neighborhood Health Center (NHC) program was designed to deliver comprehensive health services for the poor. NHCs were to train, employ, and involve neighborhood residents in a combined health service delivery and community-organizing effort that could address health, discriminatory medical care, and community development (McBride, 1994). NHCs adapted this combined approach from the work of Sidney L. Kark and his colleagues. Kark was an early founder and world authority on community-oriented primary care and community medicine. According to Kark and Abramson (1982), community medicine was defined as "distinguished from other forms of personal health care in the community in that its interest is centered on the community as a whole and the groups of which communities are composed" (p. 21).

This model was not new. Prior to the advent of the hospital, health care in the United States, in its earliest forms, was delivered in the community. Even after the first hospitals appeared, the dispensaries and the district health centers focused on the needs of the communities they served. Nevertheless, this model, taking medical care out of the hospital and back into the community, was viewed as revolutionary and challenging at a time when the country was experiencing change in so many areas: civil rights, students' rights, the women's movement, opposition to the Vietnam War, and an influx of immigrants from nations around the globe. One criticism of the NHC program was that it was too expensive per unit of service produced, compared to the services of private physicians (Davis and Millman, 1983). NHCs sustained a few minor legislative assaults in the form of budget cuts and amendments but survived the Nixon and Ford administrations to become institutionalized in 1975 as the Community Health Centers (CHC) program. The failure of these legislative assaults held encouraging implications for the longevity of federally funded health programs. Indeed, the CHC program has survived to this day, with some alterations.

It must be noted that the OEO legislation and the NHC and CHC programs that resulted from it were products of their time. Not only was the economy transforming and growing in the 1960s, but there was also a sense that this growth would continue for some time, albeit with some economic sectors growing more slowly than others. In complete contrast, by the time legislation was passed to authorize community health centers in 1975, two new perceptions had come to the fore. First, health care expenditures were growing at a much faster pace than had been anticipated during the 1960s, when Medicare and Medicaid were established as public health insurance to pay for the health care of the poor and aged. Second, it came to be recognized that the U.S. economy could not expand unabated forever; it would eventually undergo periodic downturns or corrections.

The next stage of federal funding for community-level health care began in the late 1970s and continues to the present. The Community Health Center program was authorized by congressional legislation in 1975 under section 330 of the Public Health Law and later amended by the Health Center Consolidation Act of 1996. CHCs are required to provide a comprehensive array of primary care services and to serve an established number of users, based on facility size measured by square footage. CHC facilities and programs are administered by the Bureau of Primary Health Care (BPHC) of the Health Resources and Services Administration (HRSA) in the U.S. Department of Health and Human Services (DHHS). These organizations are required by statute to provide a comprehensive array of clinical medical services, including the following (Davis and Millman, 1983, p. 127):

- Diagnostic, treatment, consultative, referral, and other services rendered by a physician or a physician extender
- Diagnostic laboratory and radiological services
- Preventive health services, including nutritional assessment, medical social services, well-child care, and immunizations
- Emergency medical services
- Transportation services as required for patient care
- Preventive dental services
- Pharmaceutical services

Currently, the CHC programs are the only federally funded programs designed to provide health services to residents of underserved communities, but CHCs have had to defend this vitally important role. CHCs easily obtained reauthorization in 1978, the second year of the Carter administration, at substantially higher amounts for a three-year period. It may be argued that because CHCs were so well funded, difficulties arose. Two incidents are worthy of mention here. The first major conflict occurred in 1978 between urban and rural factions in the CHC policy networks when rural health advocates sought to acquire greater resources for rural areas.

A second attempt to radically change the CHC program came in 1981 when the Reagan administration reduced spending for many social programs and block-granted a majority of health programs to the states. Health care funding to the states and localities before the Reagan administration was offered in the form of "categorical" grants, meaning that the funding focused on specific populations or health issues, such as substance abuse, mental health, family planning, or research. Under Reagan, various categorical grants were grouped and given to the states in four major "block" grants intended to cover preventive health, maternal and child health, primary care, and alcohol, drug abuse, and mental health (Williams and Torrens, 1999). Note that block grants are not the only source of federal revenues at the local level. Federal resources for most of the public health functions are channeled to the state and local levels through direct grants from federal agencies such as the Health Resources and Services Administration (HRSA) and the Centers for Disease Control and Prevention (CDC).

Although Congress successfully rejected efforts during both terms of the Reagan administration to block-grant the CHC program to the states, Congress ceded to the concept of greater state involvement in the CHC program (Sardell, 1988). This meant that local communities interested in establishing a CHC now had to navigate two different layers of bureaucracy, one at the state and another at the federal level. More recently, in 2002, during the second year of the George W. Bush administration, an unsuccessful attempt was made to close the Women's Health Division of the BPHC, which oversees various CHC programs addressing the health needs of minority women.

Government support for health service delivery to poor and underserved communities was provided through five different grant structures prior to 1996: Migrant and Seasonal Farmworker Health Centers, Community Health Centers, two types of Health Care for the Homeless Health Centers, and Health Care for Residents of Public Housing. The Health Center Consolidation Act of 1996 brought all these different grant structures into one grant program that is now referred to as the U.S. Public Health Service (PHS) Community Health Center Program. Table 1.1 shows the original grant numbers for these programs as well as the new ones under the Consolidation Act.

The Consolidation Act has been most beneficial to community clinics that serve more than one type of vulnerable population. Before 1996, communities had to enlist limited resources to complete the lengthy, complicated, and cumbersome federal application for

Table 1.1. Federal Grant Programs Under the Health Center Consolidation Act of 1996.

Grant Name	Grant Number Before 1996	Grant Number Since 1996
Migrant and Seasonal Farmworker Health Centers	329	330(g)
Community Health Centers	330	330(e)
Health Care for the Homeless Health Centers	340	330(h)
Health Care for Homeless Children Health Centers	340a	330(h)
Health Centers for Residents of Public Housing	340A	330(l)

each of the populations they served. Since 1996, only one 330 application is needed.

Although there has been an undeniable ebb and flow to the allocation of resources into HRSA and the work of the BPHC, the 330 CHC program has been extremely successful. Its success is attributed to the willingness to design programs that are culturally sensitive to the needs of the communities they serve. This sensitivity has contributed to reductions in infant mortality, hospital admissions, and health care costs for Medicaid patients (Leigh, Jimenez, Lee, and Andrews, 2002). The BPHC provided funding to 670 community and migrant health centers in fiscal year (FY) 2000, along with homeless and public housing programs and funding for new startups of CHCs. Since the start of the Bush administration in 2001, the U.S. Department of Health has undergone massive reorganization, with many former BPHC activities subsumed under HRSA or eliminated outright. Nevertheless, CHCs remain a very strong program. In addition to ongoing expansion and additions to the health center system, appropriations in FY 2002 of $1.3 billion were increased to $1.62 billion by FY 2004, an increase of more than $112 million over FY 2003. Information on the HRSA budget and appropriations, including funding for the Community Health Center Program, can be found at the BPHC Web site (http://www.hrsa.gov/budget.htm).

Although the CHC program was designed to be operated by nonprofit community organizations, this is not always the case. Some poor and minority communities have been able to build leadership and power via the federally funded community health center program (Schlesinger, 1988), but the reality is that federal, state, and city decision makers feel a greater degree of comfort in granting 330 funding to a partnership between municipal or voluntary hospitals and nonprofit community-based organizations. This provides federal agencies with a greater measure of security based on the fiscal management "expertise" of hospitals compared to new and untried community groups. At the same time, this arrangement also provides hospitals with an additional source of revenue.

Therefore, when a not-for-profit community-based organization seeks federal funding to operate a 330 facility, it is usually instructed to partner with a local hospital. In a majority of cases, the hospital is ultimately the entity that contracts with the DHHS to provide health services, manages the 330 funding, provides the physicians and the medical oversight, and bills and collects from Medicare, Medicaid, and any third-party commercial payers.

In essence, the CBHO serves more as a sponsor by lending its name and credibility in the community, and in some unusual instances, a resident leader may obtain a seat on the governing board of the parent hospital or health center network. These restrictions greatly inhibit the ability of many community-based organizations to develop freestanding CHCs without partnering with a hospital or large mainstream agency with ties to federal, state, and city health policy and decision makers. On occasion, equitable partnerships between communities and large health care entities can be negotiated. Their success depends on development of an organizational framework for those partnerships that will support the growth and sustainability of the partnering CBHOs to respond to community health needs.

Organizational Framework: The Development and Growth of CBHOs

Although by their very nature, CBHOs are a response to local health needs, the federal programs discussed in the preceding section have been providing health care services at the local level for more than thirty years. These national policy decisions were eventually coupled with state-level policies to provide support for health services at the neighborhood or community level. More recently, because of increasing demographic diversity in the United States, small steps are being taken by federal health agencies to focus on specific populations for targeted health services based on levels of need. Unquestionably, these policies represent a significant level of long-term recognition of the need for community-based health service delivery. These federal and state efforts notwithstanding, the fact remains that health care for the poor in the United States has traditionally been the responsibility of government at the local level.

The Case for Development of CBHOs

City-level departments of health and other local authorities are cognizant of the need to address neighborhood or community health needs. However, they operate as part of city or local governments, where efforts to maintain or increase the budget for safety and protective services such as police and firefighters have higher priority and wider appeal than health care for the poor and uninsured. Unfortunately, because funding is not infinite, this often means that these governments are caught in a bind with regard to achieving their mission to provide ambulatory or primary preventive care services for their poor and uninsured residents.

In the depressed fiscal environment of the mid-1970s, most cities were forced to cut budgets in almost every area and did so relentlessly in the area of health care for the poor. As an alternative, local governments sometimes encouraged development of local community health centers initially funded under the authority of section 330 of the Public Health Law and later amended by the Health Center Consolidation Act. The BPHC Web site indicates that in 1979, there were 190 community health centers in urban areas around the country that were federally funded 330 centers, and as of FY 2000, there were 670. Though the number of CHCs has certainly grown, it is important to note that CBOs interested in providing health services to meet the needs of their communities have not always been able to qualify for CHC funding.

Origins of CBHOs

Many CBHOs grow out of the civic and political efforts of community groups and leaders. How these groups and individuals manage to develop their CBHOs is by first establishing political alliances with their elected officials and partnerships with existing health providers such as hospitals or health center networks. Through their relationships in the community, these groups and individuals tend to develop organizations that initially start out as social support agencies that provide health outreach and education while advocating for the poor, uninsured, underinsured, and immigrants and connecting them to available health services. Some of these CBHOs eventually go on to become federally funded CHCs.

Essentially, the economic, political, and social climate of the period from the 1950s to the 1980s in the United States and around the world gave rise to CBHOs. During this time, the United States experienced a convulsion from the ultraconservatism prevalent after World War II and the 1950s to the liberalism of the 1960s, followed by a return to conservatism with the election of President Nixon in 1969. Nixon started the process of unraveling the War on Poverty program, developed to combat economic deprivations long endured by the poor, on two fronts: through federal cuts in social spending and through tax policies, which further enriched individuals in the top 10 percent income group throughout the world.

This same thirty-year period also saw increasing interest around the world and among some groups in the United States in a radically different model of health service delivery that relied on primary care, health promotion, and disease prevention rather than on hospital-based care. To a large extent, this interest was being spurred by the World Health Organization (WHO) as part of its global vision to achieve "health care for all" by 2000. In an effort to realize this vision, WHO convened a worldwide health conference in Alma Ata in 1978. Delegates from 134 nations gathered at the conference and agreed, on behalf of their countries, to focus on primary care as the major strategy for health care delivery, increase community participation in health care planning, and make health care more accessible for everyone than it had been in the past. Only later did it become clear that while delegates from the United States and several other countries were pledging to support the provisions of Alma Ata, their increasingly conservative governments were busy cutting even deeper into health care spending for the poor and uninsured.

In the midst of this worldwide, unreceptive political and economic climate, Sidney and Emily Kark and their colleagues seized a small window of opportunity, opened briefly by the apartheid government, and began to develop health centers in South Africa in the mid-1950s, based on the principles of community-oriented primary care. The civil rights movement, with its principles of community empowerment and political and economic equity that later led to the War on Poverty, opened a much bigger window in the United States in the 1960s, which Dr. John Hatch and his colleagues used to pioneer the development of CBHOs, based on the model of the black church. The North Bolivar County Health Council (NBCHC) in Bolivar county in the Mississippi Delta developed the first group of community health center–affiliated CBHOs, which were chartered as a community development corporation. Today NBCHC owns and operates the Delta Health Center in Mississippi and the North Bolivar County Farm Cooperative, among other health centers. During the 1960s and early 1970s, Eugenia Eng and Theodore Parrish were among some of Dr. Hatch's colleagues who assisted in the pioneering work of developing the early CBHOs in urban and rural African American communities in the United States (Geiger, 2002; Hatch and Eng, 1984; Hatch, 1969).

Growth of CBHOs

The United States of the 1980s was politically conservative, and it was clear that few provisions would be made to care for the health of the poor. Given the tone of that environment, it is understandable that the development of community-based health organizations, with or without federal funding, was inevitable. Although some CBHOs are indeed federally funded 330 programs, based on the definition provided earlier, some may not provide primary care or clinical services. Those CBHOs are eligible for various types of support from local and state governments to provide a broad range of health, mental health, and health-related care, including social and support services. They also qualify for state or federal categorical grants, many of which are used to provide specialty services, such as outreach and education for maternal child health, HIV/

AIDS, and other health-related nonclinical services, targeting distinct subgroups, which varies tremendously among these clinics.

Since the late 1970s, there has been steady growth of CBOs in the United States. There may now be more than one million of them in the country; the exact number is unknown. What is known is that significant numbers of them have been established with the mission to focus exclusively on health or health-related issues. The very development of increasing numbers of CBOs and CBHOs—some of them organized by newly arrived immigrant groups, communities of color, or poor to middle-income communities and many of them established to meet health and other basic needs—at this particular juncture in U.S. history is significant, for three reasons. First, we know that the development of organizations by any group of people for the purpose of addressing their specific concerns is indicative of a structural failure by the larger society to respond to those needs (Bayne Smith, 1996a). Second, the capacity to build organizations is a sign of political maturity and readiness on the part of the organizing groups to negotiate with mainstream groups from a position of power. Third and most important is the willingness of many of the new community-based organizations to function as instruments of social change in a diverse and multicultural society (Bayne Smith, 1996a).

During the past thirty years, there has been an increase in the number of not only federally funded CHCs but also CBHOs. CBHOs tend to be nonprofit organizations that are developed with or without federal funding and established as independent clinics or community-based organizations. CBHOs developed more recently than the CHCs, often as a result of dissatisfaction with the cost, quality, or cultural insensitivity of local public and private health care providers. Eventually, some CBHOs move to become federally funded 330 clinics, but some retain their independence out of a belief that they provide a necessary alternative mode of service delivery (Davis and Millman, 1983).

Health Services and the Nonprofit Sector

A 2002 study of nonprofit organizations and services in New York City's neighborhoods, by Wolpert and Seley, indicates that in 1989, there were approximately 20,000 nonprofits in the city. As of May 2000, there were 27,474 registered nonprofits, of which 9,078 were reporting public charities that file annual reports to the IRS. The other 18,196 nonprofits were amalgams of private foundations, religious organizations, large specialized organizations, and other entities. This study is significant because New York City has the largest and most diverse concentration of nonprofits of any city in the nation and provides an opportunity to look at the full spectrum of nonprofits, by sector, from small mutual benefit organizations to the operational headquarters of international organizations such as the International Rescue Committee and Planned Parenthood. The Wolpert and Seley study provides data on all organizations in the health sector in New York City, including large hospitals. This information is especially important in explaining the growth of CBHOs, for several reasons:

- Though not the largest in terms of number of organizations, health is the most heavily funded of all the nonprofit sectors.
- The health sector provides a higher percentage (85 percent) of full-time employment than any other sector.
- Nonprofit expenditures in New York City totaled approximately $40 billion in 2000, of which $20 billion was in the health sector.
- The greatest increases in New York City health services in the years 2000–2002 were in terms of age for children and teens and in terms of ethnicity for Hispanics.

Distinctions Between CBHOs and CHCs

CBHOs and CHCs are more different than they are similar. The similarity of CBHOs and the federally funded CHCs begins and ends with the fact that they are both focused on primary rather than acute or institutional care. Over the course of the past century, as we moved from the old dispensaries to the current migrant and community health centers, the Western biomedical model has provided the organizational framework for service delivery. This linear model has consistently delivered technological advances in medical care. Subsequent to the Flexner Report that led to the reorganization and redirection of the biomedical model, it became and remains today the driving engine of the entire U.S. health care industry. As such, it has enjoyed hegemonic status for nearly a century. Needless to say, it is also the most powerful force behind the

Exhibit 1.1.   Linear Flow of CHCs and the Biomedical Model.

Policymakers and health professionals often use a top-down, linear approach in which decision making regarding design and implementation of services is focused at the highest professional levels and usually does not include community input. Within that linear decision making model, decisions tend to be made in the following order:

1. Facility size
2. Number of clinics
3. Structure of operations
4. Staffing levels
5. Percentage of insured and uninsured to be served
6. Type and frequency of clinic programs and sessions to be offered
7. Hours of operation
8. Service modality: disease diagnosis and treatment

---

organization and operation of government-funded CHCs as depicted in Exhibit 1.1.

In contrast, the development, organization, and operation of CBHOs start out not from the dictates of the industry but as a response to health needs of the community. A major distinguishing characteristic of CBHOs, compared to CHCs, is that they strive to deliver a more holistic set of services based on the biopsychosocial health care model. In this approach, CBHOs tend to plan and deliver services using a more resident-responsive, if not resident-led, approach that pays careful attention to the whole individual, including cultural and community influences. This model, though effective, does not receive the full support it needs from government or private funders, who tend to focus more on specific health issues or specific populations with health problems rather than addressing the underlying causes. Another important distinction is that unlike CHCs, not all CBHOs provide primary care services. When the CBHO delivers primary care or when the CBHO is also a CHC, a medical director is of course required, but often a significant level of service is provided by nurse practitioners or physician assistants.

Probably the most distinguishing difference between CHCs and CBHOs comes from the recognition by CBHOs that health care services to vulnerable populations such as the rural or urban poor and underserved communities must include capacity for outreach and education. For certain populations, it is first necessary to promote access to and use of services before underserved populations can avail themselves of mainstream health services. Probably the most important distinction that even managed care companies have only recently come to terms with is that it is not effective to offer primary care services to underserved populations facing multiple problems without also offering case management and social support services. Figure 1.1 depicts the essential ingredients that set CBHOs apart from CHC and more mainstream forms of health services delivery.

Creating a Structure for CBHOs

Development of an organizational framework, whether it is for small CBHOs or large for-profit organizations, is best discussed as a series of steps. The first and most important step for any group interested in establishing a CBHO is the development of a clearly thoughtout, long-term vision for the organization. The next step is the preparation of an organizational mission statement. The mission statement is crucial. Everything the organization does must flow from and be in concert with its mission statement, including the organization's goals, objectives, strategies, and espoused values. Once these aspects of the mission are clear and have been precisely articulated, they must then be used to design an organizational structure that will permit the organization to function as a physical entity established to carry out its specific mission.

Although the framework and structures of organizations vary, most CBHOs tend to be nonprofits and as such usually have a governance structure in which there is a board of directors with financial and policy oversight (see Figure 1.2 for an example). The executive director position reports to the board of directors or trustees and also makes the day-to-day decisions regarding the operation of the organization, usually with input from the managerial staff. Whether management-level staff are required depends on the size, mission, and budget of the organization; these individuals report to the executive director. Direct line staff and clerical support staff have ongoing hands-on contact and provide direct services to the population being served.

To establish their legal identity, most CBHOs become incorporated as a not-for-profit entity and thereby obtain tax-exempt status.

Figure 1.1. Community Health Partnerships:
Collective, Resident-Responsive Decision Making.

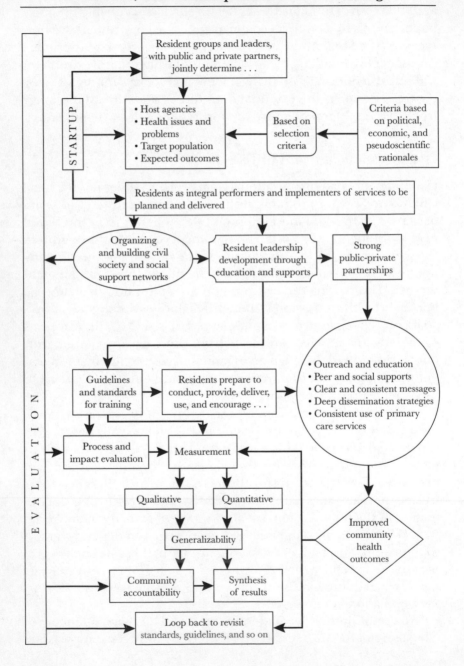

Figure 1.2. Organizational Governance Structure

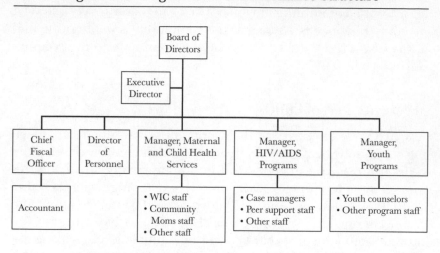

In most instances, these steps are also prerequisites for attracting public or private funds. Funding sources are reluctant to contribute to unincorporated entities that are not tax-exempt for reasons of accountability. Nonprofits are required to have boards of directors that are legally required to provide financial oversight as well as policy and managerial oversight in some instances. This structure provides assurances to the community, who in the case of federal 330–funded CBHOs must hold at least 51 percent of the seats on the board, that the community's voice will be heard and its needs met. It also provides assurances to funders that sound financial and management procedures will be put in place to ensure effective operation of the CBHO.

Primary Role of CBHOs: Responding to Community Health Concerns

Unlike community clinics, outpatient health centers, or even federally funded CHCs, CBHOs are developed essentially as a response to identified community health concerns. Consequently, as noted earlier, not all CBHOs provide primary care services. The roles and functions CBHOs are designed to fulfill depend on the needs of the community they are founded to serve. As a result, the primary role of every CBHO is to be fully aware of the health issues and concerns of the community in which it is located and to work toward meeting those needs. As long as the community is well represented at the board level, the CBHO is held accountable to the community it serves.

Major Functions of CBHOs

As CBHOs seek to carry out their most important function of meeting community health needs, they must simultaneously develop the skills and resources needed to function as strong advocates. Although these two functions are intertwined, it is highly unlikely that a CBHO that does not engage in advocacy will be able to attract the resources needed to provide health services. Advocating for improved health outcomes has to occur on multiple levels, making use of all the modern tools of communication and social action. Health advocacy must ideally start within the community being served, through education for neighborhood residents and information sharing to help the community adopt healthy behaviors. At the same time, advocacy must also extend outward. Some of the more critical external advocacy functions include lobbying policymakers to develop and implement health policy that is beneficial to the community, cultivating relationships with public sources and private philanthropies to obtain required resources to address community health needs, and developing partnerships with other health organizations, from large hospitals to other CBHOs, in order to create and sustain programs and services to improve health outcomes.

The CBHO Partnership Opportunity

Improved health is a product of social action, not just medical care. Communication and involvement of all sectors of the society are therefore key concepts that must be clearly understood and pragmatically exploited. Whether responding to community health concerns or serving as health advocates, CBHOs are essential partners in the spectrum of health care delivery, and they provide a unique opportunity for partnership with progressive organizations seeking to improve health delivery and consumption and health outcomes for diverse communities around the country. Mainstream health organizations benefit greatly from partnerships with CBHOs, as the mainstream organizations gain access to new market segments consisting of groups traditionally served by CBHOs. These are groups that mainstream organizations have difficulty reaching outside of urgent or emergent situations. One mutually advantageous partnership would be between CBHOs and the national movement of Physicians for a National Health Program (PNHP), for example. PNHP members are physicians who are active across the spectrum of medical endeavors, from primary care doctors and surgeons to public health specialists, psychiatrists, and administrators who work in hospitals, clinics, private practice, HMOs, and public agencies. The PNHP vision is for a national health program that is federally mandated but administered at the state and local levels. It would be a single-payer public plan covering all medically necessary services from acute to long-term care and prescription drugs. The PNHP plan provided in partnership with CBHOs using a combination of Western medicine and delivered in culturally acceptable formats would provide the United States with a strategy for eliminating health disparities. At the very least, partnerships between CBHOs and local PNHP groups hold promise for joint advocacy efforts to improve community health outcomes.

Key Points

- Higher mortality and morbidity from treatable and preventable diseases are concentrated among people of color because in the United States, a much higher percentage of nonwhite residents than white residents live in poverty.
- Government support for health care for the poor and the uninsured is a political minefield in which the ebb and flow of resources depends to a large extent on the amount of political advocacy being done by interest groups, policy networks, and other interlocutors at different historical periods. The response from poor and immigrant communities across the country has been a large increase in CBHOs developed by and in partnership with community residents. These CBHOs seek to address health issues identified by residents, with programs and methods designed with resident input.

- The development of resident-led CBHOs in the past two decades is a direct outcome of the socioeconomic and political climate in the United States in which the larger society failed to respond to the health needs of immigrants and the poor. Therefore, marginalized groups had to develop the political maturity to advocate on their own behalf and to function as instruments of social change.
- Policy options with a greater likelihood of eliminating health disparities are unlikely to come from traditional health professionals and their organizations or from the usual policymakers.

Study Questions

1. Historically, how has health care policy developed in the United States, and what aspects of the current health care system continue to foster the development of CBHOs?
2. Trace the evolution of community health care from dispensaries to CHCs and CBHOs. Then, based on the distinctions between CHCs and CBHOs, identify which of these entities would work best in your community.
3. What are some effective strategies that CBHOs should put in place to meet the health needs of their communities?

References

Axtell, J. *The Indian Peoples of Eastern America: A Documentary History of the Sexes.* New York: Oxford University Press, 1981.

Bayne Smith, M. A. "Ethnic Organizations and the Politics of Multiculturalism: The Case of Caribbean Americans." In J. Stanfield III (ed.), *Research in Social Policy.* Vol. 4. Greenwich, Conn.: JAI Press, 1996a.

Bayne Smith, M. A. "Health and Women of Color: A Contextual Overview." In M. A. Bayne-Smith (ed.), *Race, Gender, and Health.* Thousand Oaks, Calif.: Sage, 1996b.

Bayne Smith, M. A., Graham, Y. J., Mason, M. A., and Drossman, M. "Disparities in Infant Mortality Among Selected Ethnic Groups in New York City." *Journal of Immigrant and Refugee Services,* 2004, *2*(3–4).

Bayne Smith, M. A., and others. "Improvements in Heart Health Behaviors and Reduction in Coronary Artery Disease Risk Factors in Urban Teenaged Girls Through a School-Based Intervention: The PATH Program." *American Journal of Public Health,* 2004, *94,* 1538–1543.

Berkman, L. F., and Syme, S. L. "Social Networks, Host Resistance, and Mortality: A Nine-Year Follow-Up Study of Alameda County Residents." *American Journal of Epidemiology*, 1979, *109*, 186–204.

Betten, N., and Austin, M. J. *The Roots of Community Organizing, 1917–1939.* Philadelphia: Temple University Press, 1990.

Brunner, E. J. "Toward a New Social Biology." In L. F. Berkman and I. Kawachi (eds.), *Social Epidemiology.* New York: Oxford University Press, 2000.

Byrd, W. M., and Clayton, L. A. "The African-American Cancer Crisis: Part II. A Prescription." *Journal of Health Care for the Poor and the Underserved*, 1993, *4*, 102–116.

Capra, F. *The Turning Point: Science, Society, and the Rising Culture.* New York: Simon & Schuster, 1982.

Centers for Disease Control and Prevention and National Center for Health Statistics. *Health, United States.* Atlanta: Centers for Disease Control and Prevention and National Center for Health Statistics, 2003.

Chadwick, E. *The Sanitary Conditions of the Labouring Population of Great Britain.* Edinburgh: Edinburgh University Press, 1965. (Originally published 1842).

Coleman, J. S. "Social Capital in the Creation of Human Capital." *American Journal of Sociology*, 1988, *94* (suppl.), S95–S120.

Cottingham, J. *Philosophy and the Good Life: Reason and the Passions in Greek, Cartesian, and Psychoanalytic Ethic.* New York: Cambridge University Press, 1998.

Davis, K., and Millman, M. *Health Care for the Urban Poor: Directions for Policy.* Lanham, Md.: Rowman & Littlefield, 1983.

Duffy, J. A. *History of Public Health in New York City, 1866–1966.* New York: Russell Sage Foundation, 1974.

Dye, T. R., and Renick, J. "Political Power and City Jobs: Determinants of Minority Employment." *Social Science Quarterly*, 1981, *62*, 475–486.

Ehrenreich, B., and English, D. *Complaints and Disorders: The Sexual Politics of Sickness.* New York: Feminist Press, 1973.

Engels, F. *The Condition of the Working Class in England.* Harmondsworth, England: Penguin, 1987. (Originally published 1845.)

Flexner, A. *Medical Education in the United States and Canada: A Report to the Carnegie Foundation for the Advancement of Teaching.* Boston: Merrymount Press, 1910.

Foss, L., and Rothenberg, K. *The Second Medical Revolution: From Bio-Medicine to Info-Medicine.* Boston: New Science Library–Shambhala, 1987.

Freudenberg, N. *Not in Our Backyards: Community Action for Health and the Environment.* New York: Monthly Review Press, 1984.

Fruchter, R., Boyce, J., and Hunt, M. "Missed Opportunities for Early Diagnosis of Cancer of the Cervix." *American Journal of Public Health,* 1980, *70,* 418–420.

Fruchter, R., and others. "Invasive Cancer of Cervix: Failure in Prevention. II. Delays in Diagnosis." *New York State Journal of Medicine,* 1980, *80,* 913–916.

Gamble, V. N. "Under the Shadow of Tuskegee: African Americans and Health Care." In T. A. La Viest (ed.), *Race, Ethnicity, and Health.* San Francisco: Jossey-Bass, 2002.

Garrett, L. *Betrayal of Trust: The Collapse of Global Public Health.* New York: Hyperion, 2000.

Geiger, J. "Community-Oriented Primary Care: A Path to Community Development." *American Journal of Public Health,* 2002, *92*(11), 1713–1716.

Green, L. W., and Ottoson, J. M. *Community Health.* (7th ed.) St. Louis, Mo.: Mosby, 1994.

Gregory, S. "Afro-Caribbean Religions in New York City." In C. R. Sutton and E. M. Chaney (eds.), *Caribbean Life in New York City: Sociocultural Dimensions.* New York: Center for Migration Studies, 1987.

Hatch, J. "Community Development in a Rural Health Center." *Hospitals: Journal of the American Hospital Association,* 1969, p. 43.

Hatch, J., and Eng, E. "Community Participation and Control, or Control of Community Participation." In V. Sidel and R. Sidel (eds.), *Reforming Medicine: Lessons of the Last Quarter Century.* New York: Pantheon Books, 1984, 223–245.

Holmes, L. J. "African American Midwives in the South." In P. S. Eakins (ed.), *The American Way of Birth.* Philadelphia: Temple University Press, 1986.

Hopkins, J. W. *The Eradication of Smallpox: Organizational Learning and Innovation in International Health.* Boulder, Colo.: Perseus Books, 1989.

Institute of Medicine. *Unequal Treatment: Confronting Racial and Ethnic Disparities in Health Care.* Washington, D.C.: National Academies Press, 2003.

Kark, S. L., and Abramson, J. H. "Community Oriented Primary Care: Meaning and Scope." In E. Connor and F. Mullan (eds.), *Community Oriented Primary Care.* Washington, D.C.: National Academy Press, 1982.

Kaufman, J. A., and Joseph-Fox, Y. K. "American Indian and Alaska Native Women." In M. A. Bayne Smith (ed.), *Race, Gender, and Health.* Thousand Oaks, Calif.: Sage, 1996.

Kawachi, I., and Berkman L. F. "Social Cohesion, Social Capital, and Health." In L. F. Berkman and I. Kawachi (eds.), *Social Epidemiology.* New York: Oxford University Press, 2000.

Kawachi, I., and others. "A Prospective Study of Social Networks in Relation to Total Mortality and Cardiovascular Disease in Men in the
U.S." *Journal of Epidemiology and Community Health,* 1996, *50,* 245–251.

Korin, D. "Traditional and Medical Models of Delivering Health Care Services." Paper presented at the Caribbean Women's Health Association
conference "Delivering Health Services to Immigrant Communities:
Perspectives on the Caribbean Community," New York, Oct. 17, 1985.

La Viest, T. A. "Political Empowerment and Health Status of African Americans." *American Journal of Sociology,* 1992, *97,* 1080–1095.

La Viest, T. A. (ed.). *Race, Ethnicity, and Health: A Public Health Reader.* San
Francisco: Josscy-Bass, 2002.

Leigh, W. A., Jimenez, M. A., Lee, D. H., and Andrews, J. L. *Resource Guide
to Community-Based Health and Community Initiatives.* Baltimore: Annie
E. Casey Foundation, 2002.

Leon, D. A., and Walt, G. "Poverty, Inequality, and Health in International
Perspective: A Divided World?" In D. A. Leon and G. Walt (eds.),
Poverty, Inequality and Health: An International Perspective. London:
Oxford University Press, 2001.

Macionis, J. J. *Society: The Basics.* (8th ed.) Upper Saddle River, N.J.: Prentice Hall, 2005.

Marmot, M., and others. "Social Inequalities in Health: Next Questions and
Emerging Evidence." *Social Science and Medicine,* 1997, *44,* 901–910.

McBride, D. "Black America: From Community Health Care to Crisis
Medicine." In J. A. Morone and G. S. Belkin (eds.), *The Politics of
Health Care Reform: Lessons from Past, Prospects for Future.* Durham,
N.C.: Duke University Press, 1994.

McCaig, L. F., and Ly, N. *National Hospital Ambulatory Medical Care Survey:
2000 Emergency Department Summary, Advanced Data from Vital and
Health Statistics.* Report no. 326. Hyattsville, Md.: National Center
for Health Statistics, 2002.

McNeill, W. H. *Plagues and Peoples.* New York: Anchor Books, 1977.

Mezey, A. "Ambulatory Care." In A. R. Kovner and S. Jones (eds.), *Health
Care Delivery in the United States.* (7th ed.) New York: Springer, 2002.

Murray, C.J.L., Frenk, J., and Gakidou, E. E. "Measuring Health Inequality: Challenges and New Directions." In D. A. Leon and G. Walt
(eds.), *Poverty, Inequality and Health: An International Perspective.* London: Oxford University Press, 2001.

New York City Department of City Planning. *The Newest New Yorkers.* New
York: Department of City Planning, 1996.

O'Toole, T. P., Gibbon, J. L., Hanusa, B. H., and Fine, M. J. "Utilization of
Health Care Services Among Subgroups of Urban Homeless and
Housed Poor." *Journal of Health Politics, Policy, and Law,* 1999, *24,* 91–114.

Payer, L. *Medicine and Culture: Varieties of Treatment in the United States, England, West Germany, and France.* New York: Henry Holt, 1988.

Putnam, R. D. "The Prosperous Community: Social Capital and Public Life." *American Prospect,* 1993, *13,* 35–42.

Rosen, G. *A History of Public Health.* New York: MD Publications, 1958.

Rosner, D. A. "Business at the Bedside: Health Care in Brooklyn, 1890–1915." In S. Reverby and D. A. Rosner (eds.), *Health Care in America: Essays in Social History.* Philadelphia: Temple University Press, 1979.

Rubin, H. J., and Rubin, I. S. *Community Organizing and Development.* (3rd ed.) Boston: Allyn & Bacon, 2001.

Rush, B. "An Inquiry into the Natural History of Medicine Among the Indians." Paper presented at the meeting of the American Philosophical Society, 1793.

Sardell, A. *The U.S. Experiment in Social Medicine: The Community Health Center Program, 1965–1986.* Pittsburgh: University of Pittsburgh Press, 1988.

Schlesinger, M. "Paying the Price for Medical Care: Minorities and the Newly Competitive Health Care System." *Milbank Quarterly,* 1988, *65,* 270–296.

Schoenbach, V. J., Kaplan, B. H., Fredman, L., and Kleinbaum, D. G. "Social Ties and Mortality in Evans County, Georgia." *American Journal of Epidemiology,* 1986, *123,* 577–591.

Shattuck, L. *Report of the Sanitary Commission of Massachusetts.* Cambridge, Mass.: Harvard University Press, 1848.

Spielvogel, J. J. *Western Civilization.* (6th ed.) Belmont, Calif.: Wadsworth, 2005.

Starr, P. *The Social Transformation of American Medicine.* New York: Basic Books, 1982.

Wilkinson, R. G. *Unhealthy Societies: The Afflictions of Inequality.* London: Routledge, 1996.

Williams, S. J., and Torrens, P. R. *Introduction to Health Services.* (5th ed.) New York: Delmar, 1999.

Wolpert, J., and Seley, J. E. *The New York City Nonprofit Project.* New York: Community Studies of New York, 2002.

Chapter Two

CBHOs: Improving Health Through Community Development

Marcia Bayne Smith

This chapter employs three different theoretical perspectives to help explain the impact of politicoeconomic, social, and other changes in the United States on community health. These theories also explore the various roles that community-based health organizations (CBHOs) can play in building civil society and in organizing and developing community capacity for advocacy. The discussion promotes the idea that achievement and maintenance of good health require community involvement and social action.

The underlying theme is that health outcomes are community-wide phenomena, as opposed to individual occurrences. A preponderance of evidence supports this theme, resting on the fact that the poorest health outcomes are overwhelmingly concentrated in communities with specific characteristics (Macintyre and Ellaway, 2000; Wilson and Daly, 1999). These include lack of access to quality care (Kovner and Jonas, 2002), lack of preparation of community residents for managerial and skilled labor jobs (Clark, Anderson, Clark, and Williams, 2000), the breakdown of civil society (Stafford, 1997), the relegation of many community residents to low-paying jobs (Dye and Renick, 1981), and long-term environmental racism evidenced by hazardous waste disposal sites that are overwhelmingly located in poor communities (Zimmerman, 1993; Freudenberg, 1984; Northridge and Shepard, 1997).

The idea that there are critical social and ecological determinants of health is not new (Marmot and Syme, 1976; Kawachi and Kennedy, 1999a). Yet for half a century, health and social scientists frowned on analysis of aggregate community data, placing greater value on research conducted at the level of individuals. The past decade has seen a renewed interest in health outcomes of people living in different types of communities, neighborhoods, and regions. Accompanying the renewed focus on community health is an emerging awareness that the more viable approach for health service delivery to communities with poor health outcomes is through the community-building and empowerment strategies of CBHOs, rather than through institutionally based care. The viability of CBHOs in delivering clinical, health education, and promotion services to low-income communities is supported by research (see Chapters Three and Four). Even when CBHOs do not directly provide clinical care, they ought to be considered as strategic partners by those who do. In some instances, the move toward partnering with community groups and with other CBHOs is driven by increasing requirements from both public and private funding sources for the development of such partnerships and coalitions (Wandersman, Goodman, and Butterfoss, 2002).

A strong social foundation is required to engage community residents in advocating for improved health outcomes by establishing balanced power relationships among community organizations and groups and external partners. Community groups and organizations and the CBHOs they develop must often partner with resource-rich health institutions or other public and private community stakeholders in the health arena. Consequently, the strong civil society of developed communities is essential because, as Labonté (2002) cautions, "the goal of community development is really to develop the ability of the community group to negotiate its own terms and to establish equitable power relationships with institutions and other public and private partners" (pp. 94–95). Within this context, CBHOs provide a valuable base on which to build, organize, and develop strong, cohesive communities that can first determine the health care and other services they need and want and then advocate to obtain them.

Central to the work of building strong social foundations for sustaining community empowerment is the idea that as providers and other outsiders form partnerships with CBHOs, they must also commit to a process of both learning and teaching. This idea has been influenced by the work of Paulo Freire (1990), which is insistent that given an opportunity to identify the problems they need to learn more about, people have the ability not only to learn but also to empower themselves and take charge of their lives in order to make beneficial changes.

Learning Objectives

- The theories used by community health professionals to explain community health and community change are a reflection of myriad social, economic, political, demographic, and cultural forces.
- Community health is multidimensional and has to be addressed using a multidisciplinary approach that requires the application of blended and balanced theories.
- Economic, social, and cultural changes in the health arena in the past thirty years have been continual, rapid, financially unsound, and unresponsive to health disparities that primarily affect poor and immigrant communities.
- Social policy, particularly health policy, has not always been mindful of community health needs and has been more concerned with containing health costs by rationing health care for the poor and denying immigrants access to care.
- Achieving and sustaining good-quality health outcomes requires access to culturally appropriate health services.
- Historically, civil society within a community is built by the earliest settlers. As new groups move in during periods of transition, the groups who preceded the new arrivals often leave, taking valuable resources, such as social capital and social cohesion, with them.
- Natural tension arises during periods of transition as new groups bring different cultures, languages, and behaviors. The members of earlier groups who remain may manage to develop a shaky coexistence with the new arrivals, but seldom

are they able to work together to rebuild and redevelop their communities without assistance of willing brokers and negotiators.

- As the new groups begin to participate in the political process, they develop strategies and solutions to critical problems such as health care, including the development of CBHOs.
- In some communities, CBHOs have multiple functions: they help organize residents in building the community's social capital and level of social cohesion, which contributes to community empowerment and development and ultimately to improved health outcomes.
- In developing partnerships with CBHOs, health professionals and other stakeholders must be willing to learn from, respect, and value local knowledge as a necessary precursor to effective service delivery.

Working Definitions

A few terms are introduced in this chapter that were not defined in Chapter One. *Community organization* is defined in this book as "bringing people together to identify shared problems and to increase people's say about decisions that affect their lives" (Rubin and Rubin, 2001, p. 3). *Community empowerment* is a process that occurs as social capital, social cohesion, and civil society are developed and strengthened. *Community development* refers to the community empowerment that is the result of both community organization and community building.

Theoretical Perspectives

One of the methods used for thinking about and understanding community health and community change is the application of theories or paradigms. Social science and social change research are shaped and anchored by fundamental assumptions or theories, tentative explanations about the relationships between and among various social phenomena, such as the relationship between CBHOs and community organizing, building, development, and advocacy.

Health practitioners and researchers who work from a community health perspective are aware that community health is multidimensional and must therefore be addressed using a multidisciplinary approach. Doing this requires the application of theory that emerges from the blend and balance of political, sociological, community organization, psychological, and communication theories (Green, 2002). To guide their work, researchers rely on various theoretical paradigms. A paradigm is a set of related theories and concepts that guide research thinking and understanding of the world (Merton, 1957). The paradigm used by a researcher will influence the questions asked, the data collected, and the interpretation of the findings.

Developing a Theoretical Framework

Although there are certainly many other approaches, three theoretical explanations—the political economy, symbolic interaction, and social ecology perspectives—are offered here as an initial framework for thinking about the effects of economic and political changes on community health and the resulting development of CBHOs as vehicles for empowering community and advocating for improved health outcomes. Each paradigm represents a blend of various other theories. These theories help explain the effects of various kinds of social changes on communities, the emergence of CBHOs, and the contributions they make to organizing, building social capital and social cohesion, and strengthening civil society. Consequently, no one theory is better than any other, and no theory alone provides the fullest possible explanation. During our examination of these three, several other related theories will also be discussed.

Political Economy Perspective

The political economy perspective is an amalgam of political and economic theory and focuses on the unequal distribution of goods and benefits, including respect, prestige, power, money, and high-quality health care, education, and other services. These various kinds of goods, resources, and services are differentially conferred in our society as a result of political, economic and sociocultural features such as race, class, ethnicity, gender, and age.

The political economy perspective holds that CBHOs and other community organizations emerge because the unequal distribution of goods in society creates conditions in some communities in which the needs of some groups go unmet. Groups with less access to goods and services must organize to increase their political and economic power. Therefore, community efforts to organize, advocate for, and develop more effective approaches to improving community health are worthy of support by both public and private partnerships and resources. CBHOs have continued to emerge and over the past twenty years have been instrumental in providing health services by organizing communities and involving them in communitywide action to create change.

The political economy perspective is especially helpful. It is concerned at one end with the macroeconomic structure of the United States and at the other end with the microeconomic impact of inequality for certain individuals, who as a result experience greater unemployment, lower wages, higher costs for health services, and high numbers of uninsured, leading to negative community health statuses.

The concern from the political economy perspective is social conflict, particularly political and economic power struggles that inevitably occur when resources are allocated on the basis of power rather than merit (Kleniewski, 2002). To alter power relations, the political economy change strategies rely heavily on organizing and building community social capital, cohesion, and ultimately empowerment. At the same time, within the political economy configuration, there is also an appreciation of radical structural theory and its use of the learning-teaching approach first developed by Paulo Freire. The use of strategies such as community building and organizing combined with the Freirean pedagogy provides a framework in which poor people can consciously work to develop a voice and to become empowered participants in designing solutions to their problems (McCullough, 1990).

The emphasis on altering power relations is critical for poor communities and the CBHOs serving them. The essential contention of political economy theory is that the groups with power in a society or community determine the rules in terms of what has value, who will have access to the resources and benefits deemed to have value, and the kinds of rewards or penalties that will be forthcoming when the rules are adhered to or broken (Feagin and Feagin, 1993). These various political and economic concepts result in a paradigm that focuses on both macroeconomic and microeconomic changes and trends. For example, the shift in the United States from a manufacturing economy to a service and high-tech information society (macroeconomic changes) was followed closely by a long-term disinvestment of poor communities by government and private corporations as a consequence of that economic shift (microeconomic changes).

Political economy theory is also about struggles for political power. Despite the democratic ideals of one vote per person, wealthy people have always had and continue to have greater access to political power than poor people do. From the perspective of political economy theorists, the establishment of community-based organizations such as CBHOs can contribute to organizing and building the social capital and cohesion of poor communities, thereby empowering them to advocate for a more equitable political distribution of economic resources such as health care. The organizing and advocating functions carried out by CBHOs are discussed extensively in Chapter Five. That discussion includes information regarding the required skill set of people who manage CBHOs and the usefulness of those skills for providing health services, which are a politically controlled commodity that cannot easily be acquired without also engaging in voter outreach and registration and community education about political realities (Minkler, 2002).

Symbolic Interaction Perspective

A major criticism of the political economy perspective is that it fails to look at the world on a micro level, through the day-to-day activities of individuals. The symbolic interaction perspective is an outgrowth of the work of the early-twentieth-century German sociologist Max Weber, who viewed society as the ongoing experiences and behavior of people as they interacted. As a result, Weber stressed the importance of understanding social norms that govern specific social situations and interactions from the perspective of the people involved in them.

Since Weber's time, the work of researchers such as Charles Horton Cooley and George Herbert Mead has examined the extent to which we draw our identity from the values instilled early on by families and peers. Consequently, symbolic interaction theory acknowledges the combined importance of larger social structures and institutions, the economic and political inequalities that are the source of power imbalance from a political economy perspective, and the social norms that drive behavior in social settings. The focus of symbolic interaction theory is on seeing the world from the perspective of people and their unique experiences as they interact with, are taught by, and learn from others. From this perspective, it becomes important to provide services in the languages spoken by clients, to advertise services in ethnic media, and to create opportunities for client input into program planning and implementation, all of which help build and empower communities.

For example, one could argue in a symbolic interaction analysis that as vehicles for organizing, building, and developing communities to engage in health advocacy, CBHOs are involved in complex interactions. CBHO activities span the very different functions of helping their community build social capital, increase levels of social cohesion, and improve the delivery and utilization of health services, all of which are governed by different social norms.

If we unpack one set of these interactions—for example, between patients and health care professionals—the layers of complexity start with the rules that govern their interactions. From the outset, these interactions are governed by two powerful sets of rules: those of the economic system and those of the larger social structure. Health care is fundamentally an economic enterprise, and hence the rules of the health care system are no different from the rules of the overarching economy. The larger social structure constitutes the other set of rules because health care is essentially socially mediated activity. Therefore, the social structure imposes another layer of complexity in the roles of each actor, which include the health professional as a dispenser of expertise and the patient as a recipient of expert medical advice. Finally, and equally important, each person brings to these interactions and roles a distinct individuality that consists of a host of different elements. These include personality, culture, race, history, class, language, and the meaning attached to each of those elements, all of which have been shaped by individual experiences.

Health professionals interested in partnering with community residents are well advised to approach their interactions with patients and community residents with a willingness to learn from the local knowledge and expertise of community members. Health professionals must also commit to sharing their knowledge about health, the development of CBHOs, and community organizing, building, and empowerment with residents using a Freirean learning and organizing model. In this model, the first step is to work with community residents using reflection and critical thinking about their situation (Freire, 1990) to develop a critical awareness of the political and economic structures and how these structures will affect their efforts to improve their health and the economic situation of their community. Freirean-oriented health professionals must expect initial hesitation, mistrust, and unwillingness to express opinions and offer input. However, as residents acquire knowledge, develop trust, and become confident and empowered, they acquire a voice and in the process become strong advocates and agents of social change.

Social Ecology Perspective

Ecology is the study of how systems operate, and ecological theory, also called social ecology theory, provides ways of thinking about how to effectively change those systems. Social ecology theory views behavior as not only the result of knowledge, values, culture, and attitudes of individuals but also the result of a host of social influences, including the people with whom we associate, the organizations to which we belong, and the communities in which we live (McLeroy, Burdine, and Sumaya, 2003).

The social ecology perspective helps explain the various community changes (economic, political, social, health behaviors, and so on) that must occur as CBHOs successfully engage in advocating to improve health outcomes. It can do so because its emphasis is on the objective of systemic change within the various social influences of family, social networks, organizations, and public policy. These changes can lead to a capacity for advocacy and ultimately for community or neighborhood control. Control in this sense relates to community health services, which is a complex activity in itself, involving many elements.

One way to approach multitiered change is through methodical, careful mapping and organization of a community, based on systems theory. Indeed, the roots of social ecology theory are in systems theory, which has been applied with significant success to health interventions aimed at alcohol use, tobacco use, physical activity, and sexual risk avoidance behavior (Lewis and others, 1996; Altman, Foster, Rasenick-Douss, and Tye, 1989; Bayne Smith, 1994; Bayne Smith and others, 2004).

Social ecology was developed in the 1960s by Murray Bookchin. His thinking emphasized principles of unity in diversity and complexity and complementary and mutualistic relationships rather than hierarchical ones, as well as active, participatory democracy, and it fueled much of the civil rights work of that historical period (Flacks, 1995). Today, social ecology theory is much more likely to be applied to developing the ability of local communities, public health institutions, and city governments to engage in development activities that lead to improved health outcomes. For example, social ecology is very concerned with a sense of place and views the loss of connection with place—family, social networks, neighborhood institutions, and so on—as a step toward community collapse. Control of community is paramount. Therefore, system change is about constructive conflict as a regenerative force because the focus of conflict is on unmet human needs and thwarted group goals. As a result, healthy individuals and communities must question the legitimacy and usefulness of the existing service systems and its institutional practices and must become advocates of change.

When social ecology is applied to the emergence and viability of CBHOs in serving the multiple roles of organizing, building social capital and social cohesion, and developing community-level civil society to engage in advocating for improved health outcomes, it holds various implications for multiple dimensions of community involvement. It says that at the micro level of individuals, community members will be involved with their CBHOs in the planning and delivery of health services and in leadership development among community residents. CBHOs are also important at the meso level, which refers to families, institutions, and systems such as schools, churches, and health and other services that are part of a geographical community. CBHOs and other community organizations are integral to partnerships and alliances, as this meso level of community includes the entities and associations that build and strengthen civil society and serve as a bridge between communities and government. It is at the macro level that the long-term process of community empowerment and development around health and other issues leads to the capacity to identify the community's own health issues, develop partnerships with external and mainstream agencies, and engage in advocacy to meet those needs. From the ecological perspective, these kinds of changes at the micro, meso, and macro levels occur in individuals as well as in the families, social networks, organizations, and entire society of the targeted community.

Applying the Theoretical Paradigms to CBHOs and Their Advocacy Role

We have seen how the three theoretical perspectives help with our analysis of the emergence of CBHOs and their role in helping to organize and build social capital and cohesion within poor communities. Next we look at each of the theories in terms of its utility for explaining the advocacy role of CBHOs.

Political Economy Theory, CBHOs, and Advocacy

Fundamentally, the activities of community organizing and building are essentially political activities that can be used in a variety of ways to improve community health and other conditions. The political economy of CBHOs is that they can improve health by organizing communities to build their social capital and levels of cohesion through political participation. Because of their political activities, CBHOs are of special interest to elected officials. CBHO have extensive knowledge of the community they serve, which is developed by forming broader strategic alliances and partnerships across the community. These relationships and collaborations are extremely useful attributes and skills that help bring all of the right partners together to promote and foster community development.

Consequently, while the political economy theory is concerned with social conflict, it views those in power less as embattled competitors and more as potential partners for community empowerment and development. The focus is less on the conflict perspective of struggling with those in power to gain "power over." Instead, the emphasis is more on the feminist theoretical perspectives of balancing inequality, which is more in keeping with "power with" and "power to" (Minkler, 2002).

Unquestionably, there are signs of change. Overall indicators of health, such as life span and infant mortality rates, have improved. Nevertheless, the changes are not uniform and health disparities persist. As a result, significant work is still required to help groups in the United States engage in organizing and taking action to improve their health. Strong structural and institutional resistance remains to negotiating with community groups who are in a good position, if not the best position, to identify their own most critical health needs and the services they would most likely use to address those needs. Some mainstream policymakers and health professionals continue to resist by not acquiring a better understanding of the experiences, symbols, or economic and political struggles of the communities they purport to serve. The result is that those communities remain disempowered while many of the large, well-endowed health care institutions continue to do business as usual. CBHOs in many poor communities represent the primary resource for organizing and empowering communities to engage in advocating efforts.

Symbolic Interaction Theory, CBHOs, and Advocacy

From the symbolic interaction view, the urgent call is for greater understanding of people and their interactions with others because interactions are mediated by the experiences, history, culture, and various other elements of individual and group reality. A symbolic interaction approach, therefore, is critically important to the advocacy efforts of CBHOs.

When the symbolic interaction perspective is applied to the analysis of CBHOs as a base for community empowerment and advocacy, CBHOs must do the following:

- Lobby for changes in the education, preparation, and racial and ethnic background of physicians and other health providers who provide services in poor communities
- Require the use of informal learning and teaching techniques for health professionals that would enhance their ability to both learn about the necessary skills for economic success and share that information with the community residents they serve
- Encourage a greater willingness on the part of both public and private funding sources to invest in organizational capacity building of CBHOs that will facilitate their involvement in both community empowerment and advocating for improved health outcomes

From the symbolic interaction perspective, CBHOs are community organizations with relationships with local leaders, other social structures, and community-based institutions and stakeholders and other social structures. These relationships allow CBHOs to foster the development of partnerships that will advance an agenda of improved health.

Social Ecology Theory, CBHOs, and Advocacy

Social ecology offers a systems framework that places CBHOs at the forefront of any effort to make health care a right for everyone and a basic value in our society. Within this framework, CBHOs provide an organizing base from which to provide not only health and other community-identified services but also to continuously involve, organize, and mobilize the community to participate in health care planning and building social capital, social cohesion, and social capital.

Emerging Theories in Community Health Improvement

Along with the recognition that a majority of health outcomes are rooted in social and behavioral attributes of entire communities has come increased attention to interventions designed to create change at the community level. Results of several community-level interventions to reduce cardiovascular disease (Bayne Smith and others, 2004), prevent tobacco use (COMMIT Research Group, 1995), and encourage the adoption of preventive behaviors (Fortmann and others, 1995) indicate that the benefit of efforts to reach large numbers of people is that it can lead to changes in community norms that contribute to deeper, more widespread alterations in knowledge, attitude, beliefs, and ultimately behaviors. In an effort to help explain widespread community-level interventions that lead to advocacy and ensuing changes, researchers are beginning to rely less on individual behavioral theory. Instead, they are moving toward the development of theories that help explain systemic community change that results from community building, development of community partnerships and coalitions, and an understanding of community resources. Many of the emerging theories are part of new applications in the health arena and so remain in the early stages (Crosby, Kegler, and Di Clemente, 2002). We shall examine two emerging theories that are useful in explaining community change.

Community Change Theory

Although many variations exist, the Annie E. Casey Foundation has used a community change theory to inform and advance its national Making Connections Initiative. That community change theory emphasizes the importance of connecting individuals and families to social networks and the larger community. And as individuals and families are connected to economic opportunities that support families and meet community needs, systemic change occurs. Preliminary measurement and evaluation of these changes continue to be conducted by the foundation as well as by independent organizations and are reported at http://www.AECF.org. Community change theory continues to evolve from the iterative process of research, practice, and evaluation, especially as it applies to community capacity for change (Norton and others, 2002).

Social Capital Theory

While the research into CBHOs, CBOs, and their community-based approaches, strategies, and programs remains in its infancy, a theory about the collective social capital of communities has begun to emerge. Social capital interventions are essentially about community change in many different dimensions, including social support networks, social trust, and group membership. The transtheoretical model, based on stages-of-change theory, has been applied to the study of social capital interventions in different communities, with varying results (Kreuter and Lezin, 2002). Other models and additional studies to test this emerging theory are clearly needed.

Applying the New Theories to CBHOs and Their Advocacy Role

Community change theory, social capital theory, and other emerging theories continue to evolve from the iterative process of research, practice, and evaluation. When applied to CBHOs and their advocacy efforts, these new theories have implications that are expected to unfold in three critical ways. First, community groups, as well as the health professionals who would partner with them, will have to learn about and come to understand the experiences, culture, and symbols that constitute each other's respective realities and the meanings attached to those very different sets of reality.

Second, all participants will have to understand and accept that the process of organizing and building community and that social capital and social cohesion cannot be rushed. It requires the involvement of a broad cross section of community stakeholders. Most important, the goal is the creation of a cohesive, empowered community with a strong civil society. This inevitably leads to the development of effective services to improve health and other conditions, including education and economic well-being. Finally, community change theory calls for careful assessment of the commitment of stakeholders to communitywide intervention as that commitment will require putting in place structures and systems that will add value and sustain communities for the long term.

The foregoing theoretical discussion revealed ways in which CBHOs anchor community efforts to advocate for health changes. CBHOs provide a foundation on which to build social capital and engage in advocacy that can lead to improved health outcomes. One common thread running throughout the various theoretical approaches is the connection between economics and health. In the next section, we examine this connection further, beginning with a look at the U.S. economic system.

The U.S. Economy

The economy is one of the major social systems in U.S. society, and its primary concern is with the production, distribution, and consumption of goods and services. Economies are specifically related to the work of those who produce and distribute goods and services. The economic system is also connected to the ability of consumers to avail themselves of goods and services. In American society, goods and services run the gamut from basic needs, such as food, clothing, and shelter, to luxury items, such as private airplanes, yachts, and large homes in exclusive areas.

Around the world, employment and national economies have undergone tremendous changes in recent decades as many once agricultural societies became more industrialized. Fully industrialized societies evolved even further into a postmodern, technologically advanced phase. The two major approaches to economics in operation in the developed world are socialism (collective ownership of the means for producing goods and services) and capitalism (private ownership). Two recent developments, however, have led to critical changes. First, as a result of the end of the Cold War at the start of the 1990s, formerly socialist economies have been converting to capitalism. Second, while most individual nations maintain their own financial structures and institutions, the economies of even Third World nations are now part of a single international economy that moves raw materials, capital, production, and people around the globe.

In the United States, the economic system is essentially capitalistic. In economic terms, capital refers to all types of equipment as well as the funds and labor available, and capitalists are business owners who use capital to develop goods and services and then sell them at a profit over and above the costs of production; this investment in production is known as risk because the making of a profit is never 100 percent certain. Capitalism is beneficial to private business owners because it allows them, through incorporation, to protect themselves personally from lawsuits and risk. A corporation is legally a separate entity; it, not the business owner, suffers the loss if the business does not succeed. Although corporations do create jobs and spur economic growth, they have also been accused of greed, corruption, and exploitation of the powerless because in the global economy, corporate success (profitability) in one part of the world is often at the expense of workers in another part (Kornblum and Julian, 2001). Thanks to the emergence of the global economy, American corporations can now export jobs to less expensive labor markets in other parts of the world.

Globalization

We are currently in what is often referred to as the postmodern economic period. One characteristic of this period is globalization, in which large, powerful corporations have come to dominate economic production not only in the United States but around the world. These multinational corporations pursue profits nationally and internationally and in so doing affect the movement of money, goods, equipment, and people. Further, wealthy corporations influence politics, governments, and the quality of life wherever they choose to do business.

It comes as a surprise to some people that globalization is in fact not a new phenomenon. In fact, the first phase of globalization lasted more than four hundred years; it began with Christopher Columbus's second trip to the New World in 1493. At that time, he brought the sugarcane plant from the Spanish Canary Islands for cultivation in the similarly warm weather of the Caribbean. Work in the cane fields proved too difficult for the local Indians, and the need for a labor force gave rise to the slave trade (Mintz, 1985). By 1516, the first ship laden with refined sugar—from the sugarcane plant brought from the Spanish Canary Islands, grown, processed, and refined in the Americas by laborers stolen from Africa for consumption in Europe—departed from what is now the Dominican Republic for Europe. International trade, conducted for millennia on a small scale between Europe, Africa, and Asia, now spanned the globe.

It is therefore much more appropriate to view the current period of global economic activities as the second phase of globalization, which began around 1950, shortly after World War II. Many of the new inventions and technological discoveries developed by the United States for use in the war were being redesigned for consumer consumption and applied to the creation of a new postindustrial economy consisting of service and information technology industries. However, this time, with free labor no longer an alternative, two other options were exercised. One was to open up immigration by 1965 to allow in newcomers who would work cheaply. The second was to relocate production and manufacturing, much of which was located primarily in inner cities across the United States, to be near the extremely cheap labor sources in the developing nations of Latin America, the Caribbean, and Asia. The political and economic decisions to move manufacturing jobs to a cheaper offshore location led to economic depression in the United States, which appeared to be borne with greater difficulty by inner-city residents of color. However, it was deeply felt in all communities where jobs in manufacturing customarily paid decent wages and could be obtained with minimal skills and low educational levels.

By the time the largest waves of the post-1965 migrants, consisting mostly of poor people of color, arrived in northern U.S. cities from foreign shores as well as from the American South, the jobs they came for were already being moved out of the country.

Those jobs were essentially gone by the early 1970s. This left both native and foreign-born low-income inner-city dwellers living in decaying communities with high rates of unemployment, escalating urban rental costs, increasing suburbanization, and a diminished tax base to pay for city services. The void created by the absence of traditional industries and sources of empowerment was filled by whatever employment opportunities were available, some of which contributed to poor health.

Alongside the disappearance of jobs, suburbanization shares some blame for the downward spiral in the cities. Domestic policies enacted in the 1950s at the federal level provided appropriations to build highways, subsidize builders, and insure home mortgages. An unforeseen repercussion of these policies, which primarily benefited middle-class mainstream group members (Rubin and Rubin, 2001), was that by making commuting to city jobs from outlying areas so much easier, they facilitated the creation of suburban communities and thereby contributed to long-term disinvestment in the cities. It would take nearly another forty years before U.S. social and economic policies would begin to address inner-city devastation and make incremental efforts to reverse that trend.

Immigration: In Search of Work and the American Dream

As American companies began to change the way they do business by exploring internationalization after the war, large multinational companies began to emerge. As mentioned earlier, multinational corporations pursue profits both domestically and internationally and in so doing influence the movement of money, goods, equipment, and people. As a result, migration is one of the areas in which corporations exert a tremendous influence because people, especially people from poor countries, will willingly move in search of work. And most immigrants come seeking not only employment opportunities but also a better education for themselves and their children, access to good-quality health care, a home in a safe neighborhood—in short, the American dream.

The United States is one of the most culturally diverse societies in the world, and that diversity has been achieved largely through immigration. The social and cultural changes, as well as the social conflicts, that are part of this diversity reflect the economic conditions at the time immigrants arrive. Since the 1880s, the United States has experienced two large waves of immigration (Feagin and Feagin, 1993). The earlier wave (from 1880 to 1910) came from Europe, and the economic and political assimilation of these immigrants, though not without conflict, was facilitated by their closer resemblance, racially and ethnically if not linguistically, to the majority members of U.S. society and culture. This is not the case with the post-1965 second wave of newcomers, who are very different in four critical ways. First, the largest immigrant groups through the mid-1990s came from Asia and Latin America (New York City Department of City Planning, 1996). Second, they come with great differences in terms of race, ethnicity, language, values, beliefs, and norms. Third, unlike their predecessors, many of the newcomers, most notably Asians and Hispanics, have come in such large numbers that it has been easier than in earlier migrant waves, especially for many of the older members of those groups, to retain their native language or culture rather than rush to join the American mainstream. Feagin and Feagin (1993) suggest that in the earlier immigrant wave, few groups held on to their native language. The Germans held out the longest but eventually learned English and adjusted to life in the United States, where the dominant culture and norms consist primarily of adaptations of British institutions. It was easier for these white immigrants to blend in and "become American," thereby gaining substantial power and status. The latest newcomers, by contrast, are largely non-European and nonwhite, and they have remained for the most part politically, socially, and economically outside the mainstream and subordinate (Feagin and Feagin, 1993).

Fourth, and most important, is economic status. The more recent newcomers are poor, but so were the earlier immigrant groups. The difference in the poverty of the current newcomers is in its seeming permanence. The earlier immigrant waves came at a time when the Industrial Revolution was still a vibrant economic engine in the United States. Most were able, with little skill or education, to find jobs in manufacturing. Others were able to either move into or create a niche in an industry (clothing, furniture making, diamonds, furs) or trade (electricians, plumbers, chefs) or in the public sector (firefighters, police officers, sanitation workers) and move collectively on to economic success for themselves and their families.

On the contrary, the start of the new post-1965 immigrant flow coincided not only with the winding down of the Industrial Revolution but also with the turn toward a service and information technology economy. This evolution reverberated throughout the entire society, having its heaviest impact on the poor, particularly minorities, including immigrants with less education. In this move toward the new postmodern economy, with its conservative brand of capitalism, the nation now requires workers at opposite extremes. At one end are those with high levels of technological skill and the commensurate kind of compensation that brings. These workers tend to come from the mainstream population. At the other end are the less educated, who tend to be disproportionately people of color, immigrants, and poor whites, who work for extremely low wages to provide services desired by the higher wage earners.

For example, the flow of immigrants into New York City from the mid-1980s through the mid-1990s was at record high levels, reaching an average of 112,600 annually from 1990 to 1994 (New York City Department of City Planning, 1996, p. xi). At the same time, the second phase of economic globalization was becoming firmly established. Most of the low-skilled manufacturing jobs that offered decent pay had disappeared from the inner city by this time. What remained of legally sanctioned economic growth activities in the inner cities were hospitals and institutions of higher education, along with a limited number of smaller ancillary and support-type service industries.

For individuals trapped in the inner city, without new skills to offer a substantially changed job market and very few jobs available with the skills they possessed, their communities seemed to implode. As those who could moved away, some inner-city communities fell apart under the weight of unemployment, distrust, disorganization, loss of social capital, widespread drug use, and the breakdown of the local civil society. The illegal drug trade moved readily into these communities in the 1970s and 1980s, offering relief from hopelessness for some and the only source of employment for others. Some poor communities mustered the wherewithal to attack the drug problem head on (Rivera and Erlich, 1998), but many simply could not. Legitimate employers remaining in many inner-city communities at the height of the drug epidemic in the 1980s were few. Institutions of higher education, a large employer in many poor communities, did not represent a source of employment for those with low skills and could not be readily used by people who were concerned with securing basic services such as food and shelter. The other major employer in poor communities throughout most of the 1970s and 1980s was health care institutions such as hospitals, nursing homes, and home care agencies. They provided some entry-level jobs at low pay. So in addition to being a source of economic survival, the emergency rooms of hospitals represented then, as they continue to represent now, the difference between life and death in many poor communities.

Impact of Economic Changes on Health Services

The cumulative effect of these economic policies affected the health of the poor in three important ways. First, they rendered entire communities in the core of many U.S. cities bereft of good-quality health care and educational services, economic opportunities, and the upward mobility that many residents in urban communities had hoped to attain. Second, unemployment in and of itself is a major source of stress and has long been recognized as a major contributor to physical and mental illness (Brenner, 1977; Brenner and Mooney, 1983). When people and communities have to exist with high poverty rates and uncertainty about work for protracted periods of time, it creates communitywide environmental stress (Carroll, 1998), which leads to serious health consequences such as partner abuse and violence (Murty and others, 2000), as well as patterns of psychiatric comorbidity that involve alcohol or illicit drugs and other disorders (Vega, Sribney, and Achara-Abrahams, 2003). The health impact of unemployment is further complicated because it actually magnifies the very stress it creates by reducing the availability of resources with which to obtain health care services (Jones, 1997).

Third, the economic policies pursued after World War II were aimed primarily at economic growth, especially the concentration of wealth for a few at the top. By the 1980s, the atmosphere of greed that dominated economic and political life prevented the development of long-term solutions to issues, such as the need to provide consistent preventive health care for the uninsured. The result has been ongoing contention over health care financing and a deepening of the health industry's financial woes, for which policymakers have yet to find solutions despite the enormous health resources government has provided over the years.

Medicare is one such area of government subsidy and contention. It is a major health resource administered by the federal government, which proved from its inception to be a boon for the health care industry. It is necessary to recall that the medical profession lobbied aggressively to prevent the creation of Medicare when it was first proposed in 1958 (Starr, 1982). Nevertheless, once Medicare became law, its reimbursement potential became clear, and it was fully embraced by the medical community to the extent that the mean net income of physicians grew from $112,200 in 1985 to $199,000 in 1996 (Kornblum and Julian, 2001, p. 33).

Using a very loosely constructed fee-for-service reimbursement mechanism, physicians and hospitals billed Medicare directly for every unit of service provided to patients. Throughout the late 1960s, the 1970s, and the early 1980s, there were repeated scandals regarding abuse of the Medicare system by doctors, hospitals, and others in the health industry. As a result, Medicare fraud is now carefully monitored by government agencies such as the Health Care Financing Administration (HCFA), as well as by powerful lobby groups for individuals on Medicare, such as the AARP.

Medicare became available on July 1, 1966, and originally provided medical benefits to persons age sixty-five and over who were covered by Social Security. Medicare benefits were extended in 1973 to cover the disabled, their dependents, and individuals with chronic kidney disease (Thorpe and Knickman, 2002). National expenditures for health care, as a percentage of gross domestic product (GDP), began to rise almost immediately following the inauguration of Medicare as both physicians and hospitals abused the system. National health expenditures rose from 7.0 percent of GDP in 1970 to double that rate, reaching 14.1 percent of GDP in 2001 (National Center for Health Statistics, 2003, tab. 112).

Several mechanisms, from local efforts to federal legislation, were used to curb the growth in Medicare and, later, Medicaid spending (Thorpe and Knickman, 2002). One of them, the 1972 amendment to the Social Security Act, established professional standards review organizations (PSROs) to involve local physicians in the overall review and evaluation of health services paid for by Medicare, Medicaid, and maternal child health programs of the U.S. Department of Health and Human Services. PSROs were later replaced by peer review organizations (PROs), but both approaches were disappointing and were not effective in containing costs or improving quality of care (Horn, 2002).

In another attempt to control health care spending, the 1983 amendment to the Social Security Act created a revolutionary method of paying hospitals. The amendment put in place payments to hospitals according to a preestablished amount per case treated, for inpatient care, using varying pay rates by type of case, based on "diagnosis-related groups" (DRGs). This prospective type of payment was fixed according to the usual and customary treatments (UCT) pattern for the type of case. DRGs and tighter regulation of Medicare payments have helped bring down the costs of inpatient hospital care.

Between 1982 and 1986, the United States made a drastic shift to a free market approach in paying for health care that restructured the relationship between hospitals, physicians, and insurance companies. The new payment structure was labeled managed care (MC) for individuals with private insurance and Medicaid managed care (MMC) for those covered by public insurance. Public and private support was immediately evident in the form of state-level mandates for adoption of MMC. Private employers are also enamored of the cost-sharing features of MC, which allows them to obtain ever-increasing employee contributions while decreasing employer contributions to medical benefits programs. The primary reason for both public and private satisfaction with this financing system, however, is due to MC's capitation feature. Through capitation, insurance companies set a fixed fee per subscriber per month, payable to the provider in advance, which makes it possible to establish predictable budgets for health benefits.

Hospitals have been a major target of cost containment efforts in health care financing. While DRGs have helped cut lengths of stay and thus use of costly inpatient services, mergers and acquisitions of hospital facilities were used as a financial strategy for survival and sustainability that resulted in the elimination of excess hospital beds. Many hospitals are also involved in developing noninstitutional outpatient primary care services in the community in response to the need for increased availability and accessibility of services and to decrease the costs associated with institutionally based care. However, hospitals are reluctant to develop health services in the community without 330 federal funding, which provides a secure and reliable source of monies that hospitals can tap into to help offset the cost of providing care to the uninsured.

The area hardest hit by the economic changes and cost containment efforts has been Medicaid, public insurance for the poor. Since the 1980s, states have been shrinking their health care programs for the poor to save money, and the way they do this is to eliminate services previously offered. In 2002, forty-one states slashed benefits to reduce Medicaid program costs (Guiden, 2002). These outcomes reflect the impact that economic and political changes have had on various institutions of the health care system. Ultimately, the heaviest impact is always on the poor and uninsured.

Indeed, the problem with almost all of the conventional political and economic efforts to curtail health expenditures is that they inevitably wind up transferring wealth from the government to already successful individuals and companies (Rubin, 2000). While wealth accumulates at the top, the groups at the bottom acquire minimal gains, if any, creating huge disparities not only in income but also in health status. Data analysis from the 2000 census provides a good example of income disparities:

> Manhattan is now considered to be the U.S. county with the highest disparity of income. The top fifth of Manhattan households received more than 50 times as much income in 1999 as the bottom fifth. Those in the top 20% averaged $366,000, those in the bottom 20%, $7,054. Average income increased $144,000 for those in the top group, while those in the bottom group moved up only seven dollars [Beveridge, 2003, p. 1].

Economic Changes, the Health of Poor Communities, and the Need for Advocacy

Most private or commercial health insurance in the United States has customarily been obtained through employment. Public insurance was available to the indigent, the chronically ill, the disabled, and the elderly, and the recent passage of the Children's Health Insurance Program (CHIP) provides coverage for all children from birth to at least eighteen years of age in most states. But the economic pursuits of the past two decades and the resulting income disparities have hurt people with lower incomes, leading to large increases in the numbers of people who do not have health insurance and as a result do not have a regular source of medical care.

The most troubling aspect of this problem is that the uninsured are largely people who have jobs. It has been estimated that 50 percent of adults in low-income jobs and 60 percent of adults in small businesses are uninsured (Kronick and others, 1999, p. 1). Often referred to as the working poor, their income is so low they have significant difficulty holding on to basic human needs such as housing. This group is uninsured for several reasons. First, low wage earners often work two jobs, which places their income above the federal poverty line, and that makes them ineligible for public insurance. Second, employers are now using strategic devices such as hiring more part-time as opposed to full-time workers in order to cut back on the numbers of employees for whom they are required by law to provide health insurance. Third, these low-income workers do not earn enough income to purchase health insurance out of pocket, because the cost of insurance, even for a single individual, is prohibitive (Bayne Smith and McBarnette, 1996).

Finally, the vast majority of the working poor, a group who desperately need to engage in community building, organizing, and development, are afflicted by an extreme and chronic case of apathy that serves as a major barrier to the organizing efforts of less powerful groups (Labonté, 2002). Understandably, the daily pressures of poverty robs the working poor of energy and time for investing in community organizing and building, but without those efforts, communities cannot become empowered, and nothing will change.

Improving Health Through Community Empowerment

According to the constitution of the World Health Organization (WHO), health is a state of complete physical, social, and mental well-being. In addition, the WHO defines health promotion as a process of enabling people to increase control over and improve their health (1986). In the United States, the health system tends not to address the social problems of patients, except for areas such as domestic violence where health systems are legally mandated to do so. In addition, the health system insists on separating physical problems from mental health problems. The lack of a cohesive and comprehensive health system is due in no small measure to the fact that the health system does not encourage the involvement of communities in planning the health care they receive, and until the system does so, health disparities will persist.

Despite health disparities and unresponsiveness to community health needs, the United States continues to spend twice as much per capita on health care than other developed countries, and with few exceptions, we rely almost exclusively on the market to determine the amount and quality of care available to different groups (Boufford, 2002). In the political realm, we continue to insist that the federal government should not manage or provide guidance on health system issues. This idea is outdated not only because the federal government has managed the Medicare program for four decades but also because it is an idea born of old myths in U.S. society about the benefits of "rugged individualism," individual responsibility, laissez-faire capitalism, and local government responsibility. The irony here is that individuals are expected to take care of their own health, but government subsidies to big business, in the form of corporate bailouts and tax relief, also known as corporate welfare, continue unabated (Joint Center for Political and Economic Studies, 2000).

The negative impact of economic and political forces on health care delivery and utilization cannot be minimized. However, health care services continue to be treated as a social activity that is shaped primarily by culture and class. And in the United States, with its diverse population, health care is delivered across culture, language, class, and racial and ethnic divisions. Language provides a good example of the cultural divide because it is the medium whereby information is exchanged between patients and health professionals. However, health care communication can be difficult for two reasons: traditional Western-based health care has a technical language that is not always familiar to the layperson, and when health care is provided across cultures, subcultures, or classes, there is ample opportunity for misunderstanding.

Class also provides a clear example. Although the categories and definitions of class may differ, class divisions are found in every society. In the United States, however, there has been historical resistance to open discussions and understanding of class, and so it poses even greater challenges to health care than the formidable barrier of language. Nevertheless, when private insurance is used as a marker for class, recent information on primary care utilization in the United States indicates that overall primary care visits were lowest for the uninsured (10.3 percent) and those covered by Medicaid (11.7 percent) and highest for those with private insurance (58.7 percent) (Forrest and Whelan, 2000, p. 2080).

The concern with class—or more accurately, with poverty—and health is supported by information from the Census Bureau indicating which groups have the highest concentrations of poverty. The numbers of the poor increased in 2001, but the people with the highest rates of poverty in the United States consistently remain the same: African Americans (30 percent), Hispanics (29 percent), and others, a category that includes Asian Americans, Native Americans, and Aleutians (U.S. Census Bureau, 2001, tab. 2). Because it has been reported that immigrant health declines after a ten-year length of stay in the United States (Le Clere, Jensen and Biddlecom, 1994), poverty was also examined by nativity. Data from the 2000 census indicate that median household income declined 1.5 percent for native-born households but 5.3 percent for households headed by a foreign-born individual (Weinberg, 2002, chart 10). Indeed, almost 25 percent of the increase in poverty since the 1970s has occurred among immigrants and their children (Kornblum and Julian, 2001, p. 239).

Persistent, long-term concentration of poverty has been consistently associated with ill health and adverse health outcomes (Leigh, 1992; Avery, 1992; Pappas, 1994). A widely accepted marker of group health is the infant mortality rate (IMR), which is the rate for every one thousand births at which children under one year of age die. In 1998, the IMR in the United States was twice as high for African Americans (14.3) as it was for whites (6.0) (Bayne Smith, Graham, Mason, and Drossman, 2004, p. 4; Guyer, Freedman, Strobino, and Sondik, 2000, p. 1307; Singh and Yu, 1995, p. 957; Christiansen and Rosen, 1996, p. 2). The implication of the IMR disparity is that despite the progress made, black babies in the United States are still more than twice as likely as white babies to die during their first year of life.

Evidence of a strong association between poverty and poor health status in general (Kawachi and Kennedy, 1999b; Leon and Walt, 2001) and specifically for racial and ethnic minorities (De La Cancela, Chin, and Jenkins, 1998; Bhugra and Bahl, 1999; Nolan, 1997) continues to accumulate. Therefore, the greater challenge for CBHOs and their partners is twofold: CBHOs must spearhead the building of coalitions and partnerships among patients, businesses, and other stakeholders, and they must do so across language, class, and other barriers. These broad coalitions are needed to build the social capital and cohesion of broken communities and strengthen their civil society.

In the process of participating in building their community, people develop "social glue," bonds and linkages across multiple layers of community groups and organizations. The social cohesion that results can then be focused on advocating for improved health outcomes. The end goal of that process is community empowerment. An empowered community will have the tools and capability to come together, identify its more pressing health needs, effectively negotiate balanced relationships, and work with partners toward solutions. The caveat, of course, is not to romanticize either the community and its goals or the process of building community (Labonté, 2002); the process entails conflict, hard work, and difficult choices (see Chapters Three and Four).

U.S. Social Policy and Healthy Communities

Almost every society consistently, deliberately, and sometimes aggressively plans for change. An important characteristic—and ironically, one that appears to remain constant—is that almost all change leads to both positive and negative outcomes. Consequently, any plan for change is almost certain to have proponents and opponents, setting the stage for conflict and the elaboration of competing proposals. It is therefore important in planning for social and cultural change to anticipate the extent to which even well-planned policies can lead to unintended consequences.

The lack of comprehensive plans on the part of government to address the issue of health services for everyone in the United States is a good example of cultural and class concerns that have had negative health outcomes for the working poor and other uninsured groups. Despite our cultural similarities to Canada (Nair, Karim, and Nyers, 1992), opponents have successfully prevailed against attempts to borrow any aspect of the Canadian health care system or that of any other country. Instead, we continue to pour resources into an ineffective two-tiered system supported by private (primarily through employment) and public insurance for the aged and infirm or for the poor. Public insurance includes Medicaid, which has stringent eligibility criteria for the poor, and Medicare for the aged and disabled. Medicaid was never adequately funded from the outset. Nevertheless, it had the stability in its early years of being federally administered along with Medicare. That ended with the decision in the Reagan administration in the 1980s to decentralize Medicaid through the use of block grants to the states, a cost-saving mechanism explained in Chapter One. This permitted the federal government to reduce its share of the cost for social programs by bundling funding to the states for a variety of programs along with full responsibility for service delivery and program administration.

The foreseeable results of the decentralization of federal programs, and the absence of federal oversight, led to predictable behavior by the states. For example, the Oregon plan basically rationed health care to the poor by establishing priorities that excluded necessary services for poor women of childbearing age (Beck and Joseph, 1990). Several other states, including New York, California, and Florida, followed suit by setting limits on Medicaid services. The Tennessee State Medical Association brought a lawsuit against the state of Tennessee because of unequal availability of health resources in the Tenn/Care plan, whose patients were primarily African American (Bayne Smith and McBarnette, 1996).

Currently, the state of Louisiana is dismantling its Charity system, which continued to operate in 2003 pretty much as it did in 1923 when it was first established as training sites for medical students, thereby providing only institutional care to the poor (Louisiana Hospital Association, 2003). The Louisiana Child Health Insurance Program (LACHIP) has been enrolling children since 1998, but physicians in the city of New Orleans remained reluctant in June 2003 to join the state's new Medicaid Managed Care program because the Louisiana Medicaid reimbursement rate remains so low. In August

2003, the state began taking vigorous steps to change this situation through development of a primary care and case management model known as community care, through which reimbursements to physician have been raised somewhat but still remain below Medicaid rates. The increase, albeit small, has encouraged physicians to get behind the effort, and they have begun to provide community care participants with a medical home.

Social policy in areas other than health have also resulted in negative consequences for the poor. One of the egregious examples of social policy change gone awry in the United States was Aid to Dependent Children, which became the Aid to Families with Dependent Children (AFDC) program, popularly referred to as "welfare." Ruth Sidel (1986) explains that the original intent of AFDC was to provide in-home support to needy children and their widowed mothers. All other women—divorced, separated, and especially unmarried—were eliminated whenever possible, particularly if there was a man in the house. When AFDC expanded coverage to all mothers and children, it continued to exclude fathers.

Makers of AFDC policy were so intent on developing restrictive welfare policy that they ignored early warnings. It had been predicted as early as 1831 by Alexis de Tocqueville and a century ago by the sociologist Émile Durkheim ([1895] 1976) that the combined effects of urbanization, highly specialized technical work, consumerism, sexual freedom, and the deliberate breakup of families would make it easier for men from all classes to walk away from their families (Coser and Rosenberg, 1976). The effect of excluding poor men from family participation intersected with ongoing social changes in the 1960s to weaken not only families but also the various organizations of civil society in poor communities. The result was a breakdown in those communities of their spirit, cohesion, traditions, and sense of community that will take some residents of those communities three or more generations to overcome.

AFDC stands out as social policy that led to unintended destructive long-term consequences, including the social and emotional development problems of children as a result of father absence (Riese, 1962; Seifert and Hoffnung, 1994), the poor physical and mental health of women when the men in their lives are devalued (Kaufman and Joseph-Fox, 1996), a breakdown of community vitality, and the loss of organizations of civil society that occurs among people who are marginalized socially and economically from the mainstream (McLeroy, Burdine, and Sumaya, 2003). The damage to poor families from AFDC is all the more conspicuous because the United States and the United Kingdom are unique among industrialized democracies in that their efforts to develop family policy have been sparse to nonexistent. In contrast, countries such as France, Norway, Finland, Denmark, and Sweden developed well-thought-out policy decades ago to protect children and provide support that preserves the entire family as a social unit (Kamerman and Kahn, 1978) and as critical links in the social networks and overall structure of a community.

In fairness, it must be noted that during the Nixon administration, the Family Assistance Plan (FAP) for whole families was introduced to Congress. FAP was designed to provide subsidies to wives and training and job skills for poor men to improve family income. The thinking behind FAP was work instead of welfare and marriage instead of public dependency for women and children. The plan was caught up in political squabbles over whether its focus should be economic as opposed to moral responsibility among the poor and eventually died in the Senate in 1972 (Mink, 1998).

U.S. health policies such as AFDC and FAP hold major implications for building community. These policies may have failed for different reasons, but they stand as solid evidence that the need is great for organizing communities and moving them toward the goal of empowerment. Only empowered community groups will insist on achieving a strategic balance in policy circles between advocates and opponents of an issue. For good or bad—often the latter—disadvantaged community groups bear the brunt of most social policy. The value of involving empowered community groups in the policymaking process is threefold. First, it is the essence of what democracy is about. Second, community involvement forces policymakers to be mindful not only of policy sanctions but also of their widest possible range of unintended negative outcomes. And third, the involvement of citizens in developing policy they will live by is empowering.

Minkler and Wallerstein (2002) maintain that social involvement and participation can increase social capital and cohesion, leading to community empowerment. Admittedly, the recruitment, involvement, and retention of residents in the community-building process appears initially daunting. The usual question is, where are the committed residents to be found? It is important to keep in mind that even in the poorest communities there exists a sometimes small but consistent group of indigenous leaders who are recognized and respected as such by their fellow residents, and they provide the social capital needed to initiate rebuilding of civil society. This small group represents the history that a community can use to regenerate its social structures. Despite the challenges of this work, the United States continues to experience considerable community organizing activity (Miller, Rein, and Levitt, 1995). However, because organizing is not always successful, it must be undertaken continuously.

Social Change: Implications for Building and Empowering Community

Various social and cultural changes have occurred around the world between the Industrial Revolution and the current Technology Revolution that hold significant implications for community empowerment and health across the United States, three of which are worthy of some discussion. Although it is necessary to talk about the impact of demographic, social, and cultural change separately, the three are simultaneously occurring events that change together. They in turn affect one another and influence health and health care service delivery in significant ways, including the ability of communities to become empowered enough to address their own health.

Demographic Change and Community Health

Demography is the study of changes in population size, composition, and geographic distribution. It is the study of births, deaths, and migration into, out of, and within a region. Demographic change occurs with greater immediacy than either social or cultural change because at any given moment, somewhere in the world, someone is born, dies, or moves from one place to another. Demographic change as a result of large-scale migrations and religious differences have also been occurring since antiquity and continue today. In contrast, the Industrial Revolution prompted demographic changes both within and between societies as large numbers of workers, primarily from rural areas of the United States and Europe, were drawn into growing cities seeking employment. This massive demographic shift meant that city dwellers found themselves far away from their traditional sources of health care and community social support.

Currently, U.S. health care institutions and services are again being drastically affected by demographic shifts in the population. One example can be found in the baby boomers—people born during the fifteen years following World War II—who are now well into their middle years. Given the tendency toward greater utilization of health care resources with age, some of the pressing health concerns at the policy level have to do with how much of a strain baby boomers will place on Medicare, hospital care, long-term and home care, and other parts of the health industry (Macionis, 2005).

An equally pressing example can be found in U.S. immigration since 1965. As noted earlier, the 1965 Immigration Act allowed the entry of large numbers of nonwhite peoples. For most of them, the motivation to move away from familiar customs and cultures to a new society where their survival depends on adapting to many new circumstances comes from the promise that migration to the United States holds, which includes finding meaningful work that pays well and obtaining educational opportunities for themselves and their children, along with less tangible but equally important benefits. An analysis of immigrant occupational distribution in New York City indicates that between 1982 and 1989, immigrants were more likely to find work in the categories of operators, fabricators, and laborers (23 percent of males and 12.9 percent of females); service (18.3 percent of males and 31.9 percent of females); and to a lesser extent in professional specialty and technical jobs (12.9 percent of males and 15.9 percent of females). That pattern remained almost constant for male immigrants through 1994. However, there was a significant change for female immigrants: their representation in professional specialty and technical occupations nearly doubled (to 30.2 percent) between the 1980s and 1990s (New York City Department of City Planning, 1996, p. xii).

The impact of this change on health and community building is twofold. First, a significant percentage of immigrant men entering the United States over the past four decades obtained low-paying jobs, which are less likely to offer health insurance. Second, while these immigrant men have not moved out of the low-paying jobs they initially moved into in large numbers, female immigrants have increasingly moved into higher-paying jobs within the span of two decades. This kind of situation contributes to socially complex familial changes and cultural adjustments. For example, instead of two-parent families, often a single woman or in many instances an older woman serves as the anchor and social glue for the family. Moreover, a "family" can consist of children, grandchildren, the neighbors' children, and all their friends as well. The impact of these changes on such matters as self-identity and perception, gender and family relations, and levels of stress have been found to have health ramifications for immigrants, especially among Hispanic families (Zambrana, Dorrington, and Bell, 1997).

Among immigrant groups, Hispanics now constitute the largest racial or ethnic minority group in the United States, surpassing African Americans. However, Hispanics account for more than a quarter (26.5 percent) of all persons lacking medical insurance in the United States, and one of every three Hispanics is uninsured (Billings and Cantor, 2002, p. 398). While the large concentration of uninsured Hispanics is clearly a cause for concern, the lack of health insurance affects poor people of every color.

It was conservatively estimated that between 1997 and 1998, there were approximately 42 million uninsured people—16.9 percent of the U.S. population (National Center for Health Statistics, 2001). According to the National Center for Health Statistics (2002), the numbers of the uninsured decreased to approximately 38 million by 2000. This decrease is largely due to changes in federal policy that extended health insurance coverage to children (both native and foreign-born in most states) from birth to eighteen years of age through Medicaid and the new Child Health Insurance Program (CHIP). No similar effort has been made on behalf of uninsured adults.

Unequal access to health care is a major contributor to the rising costs of health care as the uninsured cannot practice preventive medicine. Instead, their access to health services occurs through sporadic and inappropriate use of high-cost emergency room care. One of the more critical issues for poor communities is how to help them organize, build social capital and cohesion, and establish their own CBHOs through which the community can be empowered to engage in advocating for improved health.

Social Change and Community Health

Social change refers to adjustments in the ways people relate to each other, the complexity of which can take several generations before change is evident. Social change is essentially behavioral change that spans the entire range of human activity, from micro-level interactions between only two people to macro-level interactions within and between organizations, institutions, and entire societies and cultures.

Values, particularly contradictory values, are a major source of social change. One example of contradiction in the United States can be found in the high value we place on life, which is in direct conflict with the negative health impact produced by economic enterprises such as hazardous waste landfills and garbage dumps and incinerators. These kinds of industries are more clustered in the backyards of communities of color than in white communities, and this targeting of communities of color is a form of environmental racism (Bullard, 1993). Often these are communities where residents are not sufficiently organized politically or economically and therefore not empowered to prevent or stop environmental racism. Despite partnerships between the federal-level Environmental Protection Agency (EPA) and community-based organizations and some progress in fighting for environmental justice during the Clinton administration (Gaylord and Bell, 1995), the EPA has not been able to maintain some of its earlier gains since the start of the Bush administration.

Undeniably, some health-related inequalities have been addressed. Pressure from the women's movement, which began prior to the turn of the twentieth century, opened up medical education for women, albeit primarily white women. However, there has only been small, incremental efforts by isolated colleges and universities to increase the numbers of poor blacks, Hispanics, Native Americans, and other minorities in medical schools and undergraduate programs. Penetrating medical schools, a major organization within the health care institution, and creating a cadre of physicians from underserved communities who will return to their communities to provide health services is a critically needed step in the right direction. Despite the technological and scientific advancements available today, the persistence of health disparities and the pervasiveness of inequalities in the health system continue in no small part due to the absence of trained health providers and health policymakers from affected communities and the lack of interest or will to resolve this situation.

The political economy of medicine set the course early on, moving away from education and medical training opportunities, inclusion, and public health services for the poor (Starr, 1982). Instead, medicine turned toward scientific medicine and research, which persists today and is evident in many of the exchanges between providers and patients wherein very little real connection or communication ever occurs. The need at this time is for changes on both the micro and macro levels of the health system that would improve health across the divides of culture race, class, and gender (Rosenthal, 2002).

Most community organizing, building, and development occur around local micro-level issues. However, community problems at the local level are almost always reflections of larger macro issues. Through community building and organizing, local residents are able to develop advocacy skills to address the effects of macro issues on their local environment. Through community development, strategic framing of an issue, and advocacy, it is possible for communities to turn poor health status, which may initially appear to be a local issue, into a public issue. It is only when health problems are turned into public issues that they attract the investment and resources of bona fide public and private partnerships to effectively advocate for improvement and solutions.

Cultural Change and Community Health

Cultural change has to do with alterations in the tools, norms, values, and other mechanisms people use to interpret and assign meaning to their world, and like social change, it is a process that occurs over several generations. Cultural change occurs primarily in language, religion, symbols, and traditions. Although white Anglo-Saxon Protestant (WASP) culture remains dominant, U.S. society is actually a kaleidoscope of the many cultures that were here originally and those that have been coming for four hundred years. In the process, the whole society experienced various degrees of social and cultural change as each group affected the prevailing culture and one another, some more than others. These changes need not be drastic, as when a whole neighborhood changes from white to black within a matter of years; most often it has been as subtle as learning to enjoy new foods that a coworker from a different culture invites us to partake in, moving on from there to develop shared interests and bonds, and eventually forming a community.

Culture consists of the concepts, habits, skills, art, instruments, and institutions of a given people during a specific period. Culture is therefore actually the repository of experiences, rituals, symbols, images, and other mechanisms that people use to interpret, assign meaning, and make sense of the world, and much of what culture teaches, people learn early on, starting in infancy, through the use of language (Bayne Smith, 1996a). Cultural learning occurs through the telling of stories, narratives, and myths that both transfer the meanings of a culture from one generation to another and reinforce the meanings for the adults. As a result, much of the meaning in people's lives grows out of their relationships or the lack thereof, starting with parents and others of their culture, which is to say that meaning, depending on its context, symbolic nature, and origin, can inspire or oppress (Saleeby, 1994).

Given the early and all-encompassing nature of cultural conditioning, human beings and the societies we create are, unavoidably, culturally constructed. This is not to say that we are to be held forever hostage by our culture. Unfortunately, although change is constantly occurring, most of us fail to understand that our culture is merely a reference point and that the culture of any group cannot and must not be taken to represent the "truth" or used as a standard by which to judge or interpret the behaviors, responses, and interactions of people from other cultures.

Health professionals are not exempt from cultural conditioning. Indeed, some health professionals openly admit that doctors at times communicate health information as though patients had the same level of preparation as the physicians. At other times they go in the opposite direction and behave as if patients know nothing at all, forgetting that regardless of educational level, every human being accumulates experiences from life situations that constitute a significant body of knowledge (Read, 1966).

Solutions to culturally inappropriate behavior on the part of health professionals are not easy to develop. Cultural awareness and sensitivity training are not part of the curriculum in the majority of schools (medical or otherwise) in the country. The inadequate preparation of physicians, however, has serious implications for health service delivery and utilization and the overall health status of individuals who are not part of the mainstream. At a minimum, preparation of medical personnel ought to include an understanding that health care institutions have a culture of their own that can be vastly different from the culture of the individuals and communities being served. To address this problem, some CBHOs have been successful in negotiating educational agreements with local health professionals.

Understanding and Learning About Cultural Differences

The need for cultural learning on the part of health professionals is supported by the wide cultural differences between institutional culture and community culture. The U.S. health care institution consists of multifaceted components, including medical schools, hospitals, insurance companies, and pharmaceutical manufacturers. As part of the health care industry, they operate under the aegis of the biomedical model, with an overarching institutional culture that is passed on through training to each succeeding cohort of participants.

The norms of the health care culture demand that professionals function with efficiency and precision, often within large bureaucracies, and with a minimum of emotional connection to the death and suffering that surround them. These are, understandably, mechanisms that facilitate effectiveness and emotional protection. Most mainstream health professionals are providing health services in a culturally different community. They are unfamiliar with the unstructured, complex nature of the new community, and they usually fail to equate their feelings of confusion and helplessness in this new situation to what community residents feel when they enter medical institutions. These health professionals are even more perplexed when their scientific tools and techniques appear "weak, less effective and even inappropriate in the community" (McKnight, 2002, p. 20).

The health care system, a social institution, is ultimately a business, and as such it is concerned with generating profits or at the very least preventing financial loss while also improving health. A major problem is that often health care organizations are managed by administrators who are not highly skilled or culturally sensitive, and this places some health organizations at odds with the goals and needs of the communities they serve. While patients and providers usually come together in situations that require them to focus on issues pertaining to the well-being of patients, the fact is that the concerns of providers working in mainstream health organizations, depending on the population being served, can be completely different from the concerns of patients during those encounters. Exhibit 2.1 demonstrates some of those differences.

There are many culturally influenced differences between institutional and community views of health that are not easy to bridge

Exhibit 2.1. Institutional Culture and Community Culture Compared.

Institutional Culture	Community Culture
Health care viewed in a biomedical context	Health care viewed in a sociocultural context
Diagnose and treat disease	Experience illness
Focus on pharmaceutical remedies	Focus on supplemental remedies, alternative therapies, and ritual healing
Medical ethnocentrism prevails in institutions	Client's culture subordinate in institutions
Culture influenced by power, work relationships, and work values	Culture influenced by family and community norms and values
Non-English-speaking patients, poor patient compliance	Language barriers, lack of support services
Immigration reform and Medicaid ineligibility	Immigration reform and fears of deportation, especially for the undocumented
Welfare reform—public health insurance no longer an option	Welfare reform, low wages, eligibility for Medicaid?
Cost of prescription medicines	Mistrust of medical regimen, preference for cultural beliefs and behaviors

and affect interactions between people in the health care relationship (Saunders, 1954). Health professionals are usually culturally conditioned to expect that they will dispense expert advice and devise a treatment regimen and the patient will automatically comply. That has changed. Health care providers become frustrated when patients fail to comply without realizing that patients from other cultures may have health belief systems and worldviews very different from their own.

Another area of cultural misunderstanding has to do with class and different levels of communication, even when people speak the same language. One study found that ineffective communication between managed care companies and consumers resulted from the mismatch between the high reading levels of managed care materials prepared by health professionals and the low literacy levels of some target population segments; misunderstandings were also attributed to a culturally insensitive institutional culture (Root and Stableford, 1999).

One of the major failures of the U.S. health system is in its generalized nonresponse to difference, particularly cultural difference. As we struggle to provide culturally acceptable care to everyone, there are two critical reasons for paying attention to differences. What appears from the outside as irrational beliefs or behavior becomes understandable only when viewed from within (Paul, 1955). Insurance alone does not increase access to care for those who find mainstream health services culturally inappropriate and therefore unacceptable (Billings and Cantor, 2002). Consequently, the lesson for those who would potentially partner with communities consisting of people who are not part of the mainstream is that health behavior and health service utilization rest much more on providing services that are consistent with the reality of the people receiving the services rather than those who are delivering the services.

The idea that respecting community culture is essential to serving them well is not new. Half a century ago, George Rosen wrote, "A knowledge of the community and its people . . . is just as important for successful public health work as is a knowledge of epidemiology or medicine" (1954, p. 14). Rosen's comment suggests that when health care is delivered by people from one culture to people from another culture, the responsibility for successful outcomes must fall on the professionals. Despite Rosen's cautionary statement, most health providers go through their entire professional lives not even remotely aware that many of the truths they "know" about other people have been culturally conditioned and that unless one understands the interpretations that a specific culture has of the world, it is not possible to relate properly to the people from that culture.

In acquiring knowledge about a community, two interconnected aspects are crucial: its history and its culture. In the United States, the very people who bear the burden of health disparities are usually the poor, racial and ethnic minorities, women, and immigrants. These are the same people who have historically been marginalized by mainstream culture. Today these groups are working hard to reconstruct and preserve their culture so as to build (or rebuild), organize, and empower their communities. Consequently, although intentional or unintentional efforts to marginalize people who are different from the mainstream have by no means disappeared entirely, they are somewhat less likely to be as effective as in the past in light of the cultural diversity of the U.S. population, which is greater today than at any time in history. Nevertheless, mistrust of mainstream health care services remains strong among various groups as a result of negative medical encounters that left some communities of color devastated.

For example, the Indian Health Service (IHS) is still recovering from allegations made in the 1970s that in the Oklahoma area, sterilizations of whole tribes of Indian women were routinely performed without their consent (Kaufman and Joseph-Fox, 1996). Claims of attempted genocide led to national publicity and congressional inquiries. Although the IHS was subsequently forced to develop exhaustive consent procedures, these procedures continue to have a negative impact on Native women, who are not always aware that the consent process can take as long as three months before clearance is issued for them to receive care. The result is often unplanned pregnancies, made even more difficult by tribal stigmas and reactions that have evolved around the use of family planning services, which are still perceived in the Native American community as a form of genocide.

Hispanics are another group that has come to mistrust the mainstream health care system due to negative encounters. A study conducted by the Alan Guttmacher Institute (based on the Family

Growth Surveys) found that there was an increase in sterilizations among Hispanic women between fifteen and forty-four years of age in the years 1982–1988 compared to non-Hispanic white and African American women. It has been argued that Hispanic women experienced forced sterilizations in the United States because of language barriers and poor hospital procedures that did not require the patient's written permission or allowing a period of time for the patient to change her mind (Giachello, 1996).

The strongest and most frightening case for being mistrustful of the mainstream health system is the infamous longitudinal Tuskegee study. From 1932 to 1972, four hundred poor black men, sharecroppers in Macon County, Alabama, were diagnosed with syphilis by physicians of the United States Public Health Service but left untreated so that medical researchers could observe the progression of the disease in human beings. Study subjects were provided with placebos without their knowledge or permission, they were not provided with accurate information, and they were not given any treatment for their condition (Thomas and Quinn, 1991).

Historical and cultural experiences of negative health care encounters between people from various racial, ethnic, and class groups, along with ongoing demographic and social transformations in U.S. society, are contributing to a series of small but more numerous occurrences, leading toward acceptance of community health. Four specific new perceptions are serving to increase community participation in the planning and implementation of health services and the forming of health partnerships. First, the new level of diversity in the U.S. population has generated significant scholarly discussion and research for the past thirty years on such issues as the role of culture in mediating health and illness for underserved groups (Bayne Smith and McBarnette, 1996; Kleinman, Eisenberg, and Good, 1978) and the need for new preventive models of care that pay equal attention to behavior change and influencing health politics and social change in general (Klatch, 1995). Second, it is now recognized that the perception of health or illness varies from one culture to another and that those culturally defined standards are themselves always changing (Payer, 1988; De La Cancela, Chin, and Jenkins, 1998).

Third, recognition of cultural difference has opened up small windows of opportunity for tiny incremental changes in health services that did not exist before. For example, forty years ago, no U.S.-based insurance company offered coverage for acupuncture; today, several of them do. Another significant example is the establishment of a new unit, the National Center for Complementary and Alternative Medicine (NCCAM), within the National Institutes of Health. Indeed, a recent issue of the NCCAM newsletter (2003) reported on an initiative on mind-body interventions as well as research on the impact of stress on chronic diseases such as heart disease and high blood pressure.

Fourth, and probably most important, the impact of demographic, social, and cultural change, taken together, influenced the discussion on differential health status in the United States that began at the national level in 1985 with the publication of the U.S. Department of Health and Human Services secretary's report on black and minority health. That report was essentially the government's acknowledgment of health disparities and gave rise to the national Healthy People program's series of publications. These pioneer efforts in the United States have in turn influenced similar discussions in England (Rawaf and Bahl, 1998) and eventually led to international conferences and papers on how best to address the health needs of the very diverse populations in both countries (Bayne Smith, 1999; Chen, 1999; Williams, 1999). In addition to these improvements, the tenure of David Satcher, the first African American surgeon general of the United States, stands out for its focus on eliminating racial and ethnic disparities in health.

Some progress has been made, but underlying social, political, and economic conditions for the uninsured, racial and ethnic minorities, and immigrants have not changed. Those conditions, together with the opposing culturally conditioned behaviors of both institutions and communities, are primary contributing factors to poor community health despite twenty years of massive public and private investment in the existing health system. The remainder of this chapter and indeed of this book attends to the issues of using CBHOs as a base for building, organizing, and developing community as effective approaches for improving health.

The Process of Developing Community-Based Care

The confluence of three critical developments resulting from demographic, social, and cultural changes in the United States served to organize poor communities around health services. First, racial and ethnic minorities, both native- and foreign-born, acquired a new sense of empowerment and participation in U.S. society during the 1960s and 1970s as a result of the civil rights movement. Second, by the mid- to late 1970s, new immigrants had been in the United States long enough to become naturalized citizens. Many had managed to obtain an education for themselves and their children and in the process became keenly aware that in order for distributive policies to benefit their community, they would have to become active political participants.

Finally, the simultaneous participation and involvement in community organizations of native- and foreign-born minorities and their supporters enlarged the pool of advocates, community builders, organizers, and activists seeking social justice and answers to questions on issues ranging from education and the environment to health. Although poor communities have organized over the years around different health issues, two areas are of critical importance: managed care and quality of care.

In the United States, rapid change is accepted as a given; however, the rapid rush to managed care raised many questions not only in poor communities but also among some providers, consumers, and managers of CBHOs: Why the managed care market-based model? Why is the emphasis on managing costs instead of care? Why can't managed care address the uninsured? How is this approach beneficial to meeting the health care needs of everyone? Does it really represent progress—and more pointedly, progress for whose benefit? These questions were especially critical in 1995 when the president of a managed care company was paid approximately half a billion dollars while uninsured families could not obtain needed medications. There was no advocacy on their behalf, nor was there financial help from government (Carrillo, 1998).

Greed or fraud aside, the problem with managed care is not only that it is a misnomer. The more critical problem is its emphasis on managing costs rather than on patient care, and there is evidence that it is not managing costs very well. Susan Horn (2002) reported on several studies that examined the MC approach to improving quality while containing costs. She cited a study called the Managed Care Outcomes Project that followed 15,000 HMO patients for one year. Results indicated that several cost containment practices, including delays in appointments and specialist referrals, were associated with lower quality of care. Another study of almost 23,000

Medicare managed care patients found that after controlling for age, gender, and severity of illness, capitation patients had higher total costs than noncapitated patients. Capitation refers to the limitations on per-patient costs to be paid monthly by the insurance plans to the providers of health services. These predictable costs make managed care very attractive to both public and private employers.

Prior to reports of these studies, the trigger that would get even the least likely to be politically active to begin organizing around health issues came from community-building efforts that succeeded in increasing awareness that there were two serious flaws in existing health services to poor communities. Services were not culturally compatible, for they were developed without community input and so did not meet community needs. In addition, health institutions operating in poor communities were part of the multibillion-dollar U.S. health care industry, but these entities did not contribute to the economic development of the communities in which they did business.

Consequently, some poor communities organized and succeeded in building new models of care with an emphasis on improving community health, using a very broad definition of health. While some communities established CBHOs that would provide culturally sensitive services, others developed immigration and social support services and still others established health care services that could also foster community economic development (Leigh, 2002). (More on the process of developing community-based care can be found in Chapters Three and Four.)

CBHOs as a Base for Community Empowerment

Fueled by their perceptions about what health services should be, several communities in the United States opted to pursue the development, establishment, and operation of culturally competent CBHOs. Some of them seized the opportunity to develop federally financed 330 community health clinics as that program has survived conservative administrations, lobbyists, and other policy advocates who have consistently refused to provide care for the poor. Other communities established health outreach, education, and social support services in indigent communities with both public and private support.

CBHOs differ widely according to community need. By its very nature, CBHO development calls for organizing a community to build social capital and become more socially cohesive. The development of a CBHO may begin with the efforts of community leaders who work to engage fellow residents, health professionals, and other stakeholders in providing input. However, wide community involvement is required for the identification of health issues to pursue, the design of programs and service delivery, the financing of services, and the selection of strategies for advocacy and marketing. This process of integrated planning and effort to create change on multiple levels helps organize and build community. It has been instrumental in the development of innovative models that are inclusive of and responsive to community needs (Bureau of Primary Health Care, 1996). Throughout this process, the simultaneous development of resident leadership is critical to any attempt to rebuild the elements and institutions of the civil society (Walzer, 1992). When that kind of community participation occurs, it can be used by CBHOs not only to improve health but also as vehicles for community development (Bayne Smith, 1996b).

Improving Health Through Community Development

As with every effort to make change, some community groups choose not to pursue development of CBHOs at all out of the perception that as ethnic minorities, they would not have the economic and political clout and hence lobbying power of more powerful health industry entities such as the American Medical Association or the American Hospital Association to negotiate with powerful partners to change the system. Consequently, development of CBHOs tends to occur in communities that understand that the evolution of their vision for culturally competent community-based care will occur only as certain conditions are met. The community must be ready to do all of the following:

- Become empowered as individuals and as a community
- Develop advocacy skills and use them in advocating for improved health
- Become knowledgeable about the economy in order to effectively create change
- Negotiate effectively and collaborate with both public and private partners and other sources of support

- Simultaneously balance the delivery of services, engage in advocacy, strengthen the capacity of the organization, and develop innovative models of care

CBHOs: Contributions to Community Development

CBHOs are in a position to make substantial contributions to community development. Among their strongest assets is their ability to penetrate deeply into the community, organize and mobilize residents to become empowered by working on their own critical-thinking skills and community health issues, and ultimately to work toward social change. Another substantial asset of CBHOs created by community groups is the ability to carefully select, train, and effectively use local residents not only as staff but also as community organizers. This is a significant asset because it means that residents are able to deliver sensitive health messages to their neighbors by virtue of shared cultural and circumstantial similarities, which is simply not the case with professionals. Moreover, residents have more of a right and greater persuasive power than professionals to insist that one of their peers practice preventive health behaviors. This is known as the moral authority that one peer has in making demands of or simply encouraging another peer. Coming from a professional, the same message could be interpreted as disrespectful. Evaluations of this peer-educator model indicate that it is being used successfully (Delgado, 2002).

CBHOs also serve as a natural pipeline for leadership development in poor communities. CBHOs that initially hire community workers who have little formal training but reflect the demographic, social, and cultural characteristics of the community and are more in tune with its needs are in a better position to influence behavior change. With the provision of basic community mobilization, outreach and education training, motivation, and support in the quest for more education, it becomes a win-win situation for the CBHO, the staff person, and the entire community. As staff learn more about the political and economic systems and how they function, they become empowered by their newfound awareness, knowledge, and skills. Empowered residents are much more likely to become involved in the next levels of policy change and community development. Consequently, one of the major contributions of CBHOs to community development is their capacity to provide opportunities for both formal and informal education and leadership development across the full spectrum of the community.

Learning and Teaching for Empowerment

Clearly, CBHOs play a significant role in community health education and in community education in general. This does not all happen through formal education mechanisms. In fact, when partnerships are genuine, there must be a commitment to a process of ongoing learning and teaching, understanding, and constructive conflict as the partners proceed to organize and develop community. The work of Paulo Freire provides a rationale and a guide to the pedagogical concepts of learning from and teaching each other. In *Pedagogy of the Oppressed,* Freire (1990) argues that true partnership is a mutual process without which true development of people and communities cannot occur. This process allows both those who are oppressed by the systems they live in and those who participate however unwittingly or unwillingly in the oppression to learn of their roles in the system. Once that is understood, they can consciously begin the mutual process of making changes in the way they will relate to each other and therefore in the way their political, social, economic, and other systems operate.

Freire's concepts of "conscientization" and "pedagogy of the oppressed" strengthen community cohesion building and empowerment, as these concepts are an invitation to community members and partners to reflect on their actions, values, and situations, see them as they really are, and then do something about them (O'Gorman, 1995). It starts out with understanding how structures and institutions operate, as well as how people, cultures, and needs differ, and the responsibility that all parties—poor residents, community groups and organizations, and their public and private partners—have to health improvement and community development. Communities awakened to their rights and responsibilities through sociopolitical learning soon begin to question those who make policy decisions that the poor must live with and to recognize the strength they have in unity. That is how individuals and communities empower themselves to become successful agents of social change.

A pivotal concept in Freirean philosophy is the rejection of traditional education, or what Freire calls the "banking" concept of education. When education takes place from a banking perspective, students are assumed to know nothing and so are treated as mere depositories that receive and store the information deposited in them by teachers, who know everything. Freire recommends a different approach to adult education more in line with nonformal education, also referred to as andragogy, particularly for those who may be illiterate or who may have been miseducated.

The kind of conscientious reflection and action that Freire talks about is rarely found in most developed societies today. Indeed, one of the most widely held beliefs in U.S. society is that with a little luck, anyone can become incredibly wealthy. This belief is so deeply entrenched that the wealthiest top 1 percent continue to amass and hoard wealth with impunity, leaving poor communities at risk for a host of social problems (Denhardt and Glaser, 1999). Even though real wages in relation to inflation have not increased for the poor in almost thirty years, Congress routinely revises the tax code to benefit the wealthiest in the population with few if any complaints from those who do not benefit. The lack of opposition, in a democracy, to those types of tax laws is driven by the prevailing romanticized sentiment that those laws will serve to protect all who aspire to be wealthy, whenever they eventually achieve that goal. These sentiments are not diminished by the reality that the most predictable route to improved financial circumstances for the poor is education and that the United States has a history of uneven educational opportunity.

Freire's ideas about education are also crucial. Education is considered one of the most important institutions of any society for two major reasons. First, the primary importance of education in the United States is that it has historically been the means by which different groups in this society are either not educated, miseducated, or properly educated, and that depends, of course, on the group in question. Second, and probably more important, the highest quality of education in the United States has always been available only to those who attend the more prestigious schools. Today, the independent high schools are direct feeders of their graduates into the elite Ivy League colleges and universities. These are also the places where intergenerational transfers of power occur. Therefore, from a socio-cultural perspective, formal education—in high-quality schools as opposed to disinvested inner-city schools—has the ability to empower or oppress. Based on Freire's teaching, we know that oppressive education is at the root of disempowerment.

Pedagogy Versus Andragogy

Pedagogy refers to the teaching and preparation of children and young people. One of the best-kept secrets in the United States is that this superpower nation is plagued by high levels of illiteracy and consequently low levels of comprehension, primarily in poor and minority communities. According to the national Partnership for Clear Health Communication, one in three Americans has "low health literacy," defined as the ability to read, understand, and act on health information or instructions. This problem is so serious that it outranks age, income, employment status, and race or ethnicity as the strongest predictor of poor health status (Late, 2003).

The problems with health literacy are actually indicative of a larger problem. The United States is one of the most technologically advanced and most information-based societies on the planet. Low literacy is a major handicap that many residents of poor communities nevertheless manage to survive, albeit with extreme difficulty, destined as they are to remain in low-wage jobs. Their survival is possible because human beings are skilled at devising compensatory methods for communicating and for obtaining and sharing information. The very ability to camouflage the inability to read and write required an education, at the very least, in creating distraction. As a result, in every human group or community, individuals are educated, either formally or through social circumstances and culture.

Andragogy is an adult education theory similar to that of nonformal education. Unlike pedagogy, andragogy and nonformal education rest on the belief that adults learn better if they choose what they want and need to learn. Practitioners of andragogy apply the rules of respect, immediacy, and experience and espouses the idea that adults retain 20 percent of what they hear, 40 percent of what they see, and 80 percent of what they discover for themselves (McCullough, 1990).

In Freirean thinking, the andragogy approach to education, unlike the "banking" approach, is essentially about freedom and regeneration. Freire cautions that "authentic" education does not flow exclusively from the teacher to the student. Rather, it is provided jointly between teacher and student so that both parties are challenged to learn from and to teach each other about the various themes and concepts that each wants and needs to grasp about the world of the other so that together they are ultimately able to bring about the kinds of social change that is mutually beneficial (Freire, 1990).

In the United States, most people who have lived in poor inner-city communities in the past fifty years, whether they attended their local public school system or not and whether they can read and write or not, have managed to acquire an education. That education, like the education in high-quality schools, also shaped those who received it. It is an education obtained from experiences they would not have survived without the benefit of specific kinds of knowledge. The education that many residents of poor communities receive equips them with coping and harm avoidance skills unknown to the general population but some of which other people would do well to learn. As a result, there is a value in local knowledge that those from outside, seeking partnerships, must take the time to learn and clearly understand.

Freire's work suggests that outside partners may want to refrain from using a banking mentality that would allow them to go to the community with an already designed program that may or may not have anything to do with the reality of that community. Such a program is essentially designed to fail. Instead, true partnership works with a community first to respectfully learn from the community what the situation is like, then to examine the level of residents' awareness about that situation, and finally to generate jointly with residents some of the possible approaches that might be implemented to respond to the situation.

Conclusion

This process of simultaneous learning and consistent involvement of all partners from the beginning of the partnership solidifies partnerships and imbues them with greater-than-average potential for effectiveness and success. Early and continuous involvement of all partners facilitates a process of change as it allows community members to own their health and economic issues and to work with partners to develop solutions uniquely suited to their reality; this provides a greater assurance of success than anything imposed from outside.

The sense of empowerment that results equips community members to organize and if necessary to advocate for resources, services, and improved health outcomes. Community groups cannot do this work alone; neither can groups consisting primarily of mainstream health professionals. Partnerships with CBHOs allow participants to work on building capacity for themselves and their organizations while conducting community assessments and, most important of all, learning about community culture, health behaviors, and health practices.

That kind of learning is reflected in the words one group of South African people use for "learning": *uakana,* "building each other," and *uglolana,* "sharpening each other" (Shanahan and Ward, 1995, p. 74). Learning from each other builds community, which facilitates organizing and leads ultimately to community empowerment and development. In Freirean thinking, the goal of learning from each other, the payoff, is that this process is both liberating and empowering for all involved. It is this sense of empowerment, of having some ownership of and control over this reality, that moves people, communities, and partnerships from generating ideas to taking action that can lead to actual solutions. Without that sense of empowerment, it is very difficult to make change.

Key Points

- Structural destabilization in some U.S. communities in the past half century has made it difficult for people living in those communities to protect their health.
- One approach for improving poor health status rests on the development of CBHOs as a base for organizing and developing community and for advocating.
- CBHOs, more than any other community institution or system in poor communities (education, faith-based, or judicial), are pivotally positioned to influence community health changes

through their involvement and work with different segments and levels of a community, including residents, elected officials, and potential partners.

- Various structures, systems, and institutions are present in every community, along with different types, amounts, and strengths of assets and social capital, and these can be used for community development and empowerment.
- CBHOs can tap in to resident leadership to activate community readiness and capacity to act on improving community health.
- Community involvement and participation help identify the various roles that local residents can play in CBO and CBHO development, as well as the contributions of CBHOs to the empowerment of residents and the economic sustainability of the communities they serve.

Study Questions

1. Think for a moment about the community in which you currently live. Identify some of the community-organizing and community-building activities that take place there. Consider your level of involvement in those activities. Select two or three areas that may be of interest to you, and find out to whom in the community you should talk about becoming involved.
2. Describe some of the theoretical underpinnings of CBHOs discussed in this chapter, and explain how these theories—or any other theory you would prefer to apply—help explain the ways in which the health care system that serves your community is organized and how services are delivered.

References

Altman, D., Foster, V., Rasenick-Douss, L., and Tye, J. "Reducing the Illegal Sale of Cigarettes to Minors." *Journal of the American Medical Association,* 1989, *261,* 80–83.

Avery, B. Y. "The Health Status of Black Women." In R. L. Brathwaite and S. E. Taylor (eds.), *Health Issues in the Black Community.* San Francisco: Jossey-Bass, 1992.

Bayne Smith, M. A. "The Teen Incentive Program: Evaluation of a Health Promotion Model for Adolescent Pregnancy Prevention." *Journal of Health Education,* 1994, *25,* 24–29.

Bayne Smith, M. A. "Ethnic Organizations and the Politics of Multiculturalism: The Case of Caribbean-Americans." In J. Stanfield (ed.), *Research in Social Policy.* Vol. 4. Greenwich, Conn.: JAI, 1996a.

Bayne Smith, M. A. "Health and Women of Color: A Contextual Overview." In M. A. Bayne Smith (ed.), *Race, Gender, and Health.* Thousand Oaks, Calif.: Sage, 1996b.

Bayne Smith, M. A. "Primary Care Choices and Opportunities for Racial/Ethnic Minority Populations in the USA and UK: A Comparative Study." *Ethnicity and Health,* 1999, *4,* 165–188.

Bayne Smith, M. A., Graham, Y. J., Mason, M. A., and M. Drossman. "Disparities in Infant Mortality Among Selected Ethnic Groups in New York City." *Journal of Immigrant Health and Refugee Services,* 2004, *2*(3–4).

Bayne Smith, M. A., and McBarnette, L. S. "Redefining Health in the 21st Century." In M. A. Bayne Smith (ed.), *Race, Gender, and Health.* Thousand Oaks, Calif.: Sage, 1996.

Bayne Smith, M. A., and others. "Improvements in Heart Health Behaviors and Reduction in Coronary Artery Disease Risk Factors in Urban Teenaged Girls Through a School-Based Intervention: The PATH Program." *American Journal of Public Health,* 2004, *94,* 1538–1543.

Beck, M., and Joseph, N. "Not Enough at All: Oregon's Experiments with Rationing Health Care." *Newsweek,* May 14, 1990, pp. 53–54.

Beveridge, A. "The Affluent of Manhattan." *Gotham Gazette.com.* [http://gothamgazette.com/article//20030611/5/421]. June 2003.

Bhugra, D., and Bahl, V. (eds.). *Ethnicity: An Agenda for Mental Health.* London: Royal College of Psychiatrists, 1999.

Billings, J., and Cantor, J. C. "Access." In A. R. Kovner and S. Jonas (eds.), *Health Care Delivery in the United States.* (7th ed.) New York: Springer, 2002.

Boufford, J. I. "Foreword." In A. R. Kovner and S. Jonas (eds.), *Health Care Delivery in the United States.* (7th ed.) New York: Springer, 2002.

Brenner, M. H. "Personal Stability and Economic Security." *Social Policy,* 1977, *18,* 2–5.

Brenner, M. H., and Mooney, A. "Unemployment and Health in a Context of Social Change." *Social Science and Medicine,* 1983, *14,* 1125–1138.

Bullard, R. D. "Anatomy of Environmental Racism and the Environmental Justice Movement." In R. D. Bullard (ed.), *Confronting Environmental Racism: Voices from the Grassroots.* Boston: South End Press, 1993.

Bureau of Primary Health Care, Health Resources and Services Administration. *Models That Work: The 1996 Compendium of Innovative Primary Health Care Programs for Underserved and Vulnerable Populations.* Washington, D.C.: U.S. Department of Health and Human Services, 1996.

Carrillo, J. E. "Foreword." In V. De La Cancela, J. L. Chin, and Y. M. Jenkins, *Community Health Psychology: Empowerment for Diverse Communities*. New York: Routledge, 1998.

Carroll, G. *Environmental Stress and African Americans: The Other Side of the Moon*. Westport, Conn.: Praeger, 1998.

Chen, M. S., Jr. "Informal Care and the Empowerment of Minority Communities: Comparisons Between the USA and the UK." *Ethnicity and Health*, 1999, *4*, 139–151.

Christiansen, S., and Rosen, A. "Black Infant Mortality." Paper developed for Memorial Health System of South Bend, Indiana. South Bend, Ind.: Family Connection of St. Joseph County, 1996.

Clark, R., Anderson, N. B., Clark, V. R., and Williams, D. R. "Racism as a Stressor for African Americans: A Bio-Psychosocial Model." *American Psychologist*, 2000, *54*, 805–816.

COMMIT Research Group. "Community Intervention Trial for Smoking Cessation (COMMIT): II. Changes in Adult Cigarette Smoking Prevalence." *American Journal of Public Health*, 1995, *85*, 193–200.

Coser, L. A., and Rosenberg, B. (eds.). *Sociological Theory: A Book of Readings*. (4th ed.) Old Tappan, N.J.: Macmillan, 1976.

Crosby, R. A., Kegler, M. C., and Di Clemente, R. J. "Understanding and Applying Theory in Health Promotion Practice and Research." In R. J. Di Clemente, R. J. Crosby, and M. C. Kegler (eds.), *Emerging Theories in Health Promotion, Practice, and Research*. San Francisco: Jossey-Bass, 2002.

De La Cancela, V., Chin, J. L., and Jenkins, Y. M. *Community Health Psychology: Empowerment for Diverse Communities*. New York: Routledge, 1998.

Delgado, D. Y. *The Plain Talk Implementation Guide: Tools for Developing Community Programs to Reduce Teen Pregnancy, STDs, and HIV/AIDS*. Baltimore: Annie E. Casey Foundation, 2002.

Denhardt, R. B., and Glaser, M. A. "Communities at Risk: A Community Perspective on Urban Social Problems." *National Civic Review*, 1999, *88*, 145–153.

Durkheim, É. *The Rules of Sociological Method*. In L. A. Coser and B. Rosenberg (eds.), *Sociological Theory: A Book of Readings*. (4th ed.) Old Tappan, N.J.: Macmillan, 1976. (Originally published 1895).

Dye, T. R., and Renick, J. "Political Power and City Jobs: Determinants of Minority Employment." *Social Science Quarterly*, 1981, *62*, 475–486.

Feagin, J. R., and Feagin, C. B. *Racial and Ethnic Relations*. (4th ed.) Upper Saddle River, N.J.: Prentice Hall, 1993.

Flacks, R. "Think Globally, Act Politically: Some Notes Toward New Movement Strategy." In M. Darnovsky, B. Epstein, and R. Flacks (eds.),

Cultural Politics and Social Movements. Philadelphia: Temple University Press, 1995.

Forrest, C. B., and Whelan, E.-M. "Primary Care Safety-Net Delivery Sites in the United States: A Comparison of Community Health Centers, Hospital Outpatient Departments, and Physician Offices." *Journal of the American Medical Association,* 2000, *284,* 2077–2083.

Fortmann, S. P., and others. "Community Intervention Trials: Reflections on the Stanford Five-City Project Experience." *American Journal of Epidemiology,* 1995, *142,* 576–585.

Freire, P. *Pedagogy of the Oppressed.* New York: Continuum, 1990.

Freudenberg, N. *Not in Our Backyards: Community Action for Health and the Environment.* New York: Monthly Review Press, 1984.

Gaylord, C. E., and Bell, E. "Environmental Justice: A National Priority." In L. Westra and P. S. Wenz (eds.), *Faces of Environmental Racism: Confronting Issues of Global Justice.* Lanham, Md.: Rowman & Littlefield, 1995.

Giachello, A. "Latino Women." In M. A. Bayne Smith (ed.), *Race, Gender, and Health.* Thousand Oaks, Calif.: Sage, 1996.

Green, L. W. "Foreword." In R. J. Di Clemente, R. A. Crosby, and M. C. Kegler (eds.), *Emerging Theories in Health Promotion, Practice, and Research.* San Francisco: Jossey-Bass, 2002.

Guiden, M. "Health Care Hurt by Medicaid Cuts: Millions Could Be Affected." *Focus,* Nov.-Dec. 2002, p. 12.

Guyer, B., Freedman, M. A., Strobino, D. M., and Sondik, E. J. "Annual Summary of Vital Statistics: Trends in the Health of Americans During the 20th Century." *Pediatrics,* 2000, *106,* 1307–1317.

Horn, S. D. "Improving Quality of Care." In A. R. Kovner and S. Jonas (eds.), *Health Care Delivery in the United States.* (7th ed.) New York: Springer, 2002.

Joint Center for Political and Economic Studies. "Corporate Welfare: A Crisis for Democracy." *Focus,* Sept. 2000, pp. 6–8.

Jones, L. "The Health Consequences of Economic Recessions." In M. J. Holosko and M. D. Feit (eds.), *Health and Poverty.* Binghamton, N.Y.: Haworth Press, 1997.

Kamerman, S. B., and Kahn, A. J. *Family Policy: Government and Families in Fourteen Countries.* New York: Columbia University Press, 1978.

Kaufman, J. A., and Joseph-Fox, Y. K. "American Indian and Alaska Native Women." In M. A. Bayne Smith (ed.), *Race, Gender, and Health.* Thousand Oaks, Calif.: Sage, 1996.

Kawachi, I., and Kennedy, B. P. "Health and Social Cohesion." In I. Kawachi, B. P. Kennedy, and R. G. Wilkinson (eds.), *The Society and Population Health Reader: Income Inequality and Health.* New York: New Press, 1999a.

Kawachi, I., and Kennedy, B. P. "The Relationship of Income Inequality to Mortality: Does the Choice of Indicator Matter?" In I. Kawachi, B. P. Kennedy, and R. G. Wilkinson (eds.), *The Society and Population Health Reader: Income Inequality and Health.* New York: New Press, 1999b.

Klatch, R. E. "The Counterculture, the New Left, and the New Right." In M. Darnovsky, B. Epstein, and R. Flacks (eds.), *Cultural Politics and Social Movements.* Philadelphia: Temple University Press, 1995.

Kleinman, A., Eisenberg, L., and Good, B. "Culture, Illness, and Care." *Annals of Internal Medicine,* 1978, *88,* 251–258.

Kleniewski, N. *Cities, Change, and Conflict: A Political Economy of Urban Life.* Belmont, Calif.: Wadsworth, 2002.

Kornblum, W., and Julian, J. *Social Problems.* (10th ed.) Upper Saddle River, N.J.: Prentice Hall, 2001.

Kovner, A. R., and Jonas, S. "Introduction: The State of Health Care Delivery in the United States." In A. R. Kovner and S. Jonas (eds.), *Health Care Delivery in the United States.* (7th ed.) New York: Springer, 2002.

Kronick, R., and others. *Expansion of Health Care to the Working Poor: Lessons from Other States on Improving Coverage.* Berkeley: California Policy Research Center, 1999.

Kreuter, M. W., and Lezin, N. "Social Capital Theory: Implications for Community-Based Health Promotion." In R. J. Di Clemente, R. A. Crosby, and M. C. Kegler (eds.), *Emerging Theories in Health Promotion, Practice, and Research.* San Francisco: Jossey-Bass, 2002.

Labonté, R. "Community, Community Development, and the Forming of Authentic Partnerships: Some Critical Reflections." In M. Minkler (ed.), *Community Organizing and Community Building for Health.* New Brunswick, N.J.: Rutgers University Press, 2002.

Late, M. "Literacy Status Among Major Predictors of Healthiness." *Nation's Health,* June-July 2003, p. 13.

Le Clere, F. B., Jensen, L., and Biddlecom, A. E. "Health Care Utilization, Family Context, and Adaptation Among Immigrants in the United States." *Journal of Health and Social Behavior,* 1994, *35,* 370–384.

Leigh, W. A. *A Health Assessment of Black Americans: A Fact Book.* Washington, D.C.: Joint Center for Political and Economic Studies, 1992.

Leigh, W. A., Jimenez, M. A., Lee, D. H., and Andrews, J. L. *Resource Guide to Community-Based Health and Community Development Initiatives.* Washington, D.C.: Joint Center for Political and Economic Studies, 2002.

Leon, D., and Walt, G. "Poverty, Inequality and Health in International Perspective: A Divided World?" In D. Leon and G. Walt (eds.), *Poverty Inequality and Health.* London: Oxford University Press, 2001.

Lewis, R. K. and others. "Evaluating the Effects of a Community Coalition's Efforts to Reduce Illegal Sales of Alcohol and Tobacco Products to Minors." *Journal of Community Health,* 1996, *21,* 429–436.

Louisiana Hospital Association. *Task Force on Indigent Care and Medical Education Recommendations to the Louisiana State University Board of Supervisors.* Baton Rouge: Louisiana Hospital Association, 2003.

Macintyre, S., and Ellaway, A. "Ecological Approaches: Rediscovering the Role of the Physical and Social Environment." In L. F. Berkman and I. Kawachi (eds.), *Social Epidemiology.* New York: Oxford University Press, 2000.

Macionis, J. J. *Society: The Basics.* (8th ed.) Upper Saddle River, N.J.: Prentice Hall, 2005.

Marmot, M., and Syme, S. L. "Acculturation and Coronary Heart Disease in Japanese Americans." *American Journal of Epidemiology,* 1976, *104,* 247–255.

McCullough, K. "Moving from Pedagogy to Andragogy." In R. Hiemstra and B. Sisco (eds.), *Individualizing Instruction: Making Learning Personal, Empowering, and Successful.* San Francisco: Jossey Bass, 1990.

McKnight, J. L. 'Two Tools for Well-Being." In M. Minkler (ed.), *Community Organizing and Community Building for Health.* New Brunswick, N.J.: Rutgers University Press, 2002.

McLeroy, K., Burdine J., and Sumaya, C. "Community Based Interventions." *American Journal of Public Health,* 2003, *93,* 529–533.

Merton, R. K. *Social Theory and Social Structure.* New York: Free Press, 1957.

Miller, S. M., Rein, M., and Levitt, P. "Community Action in the United States." In G. Craig and M. Mayo (eds.), *Community Empowerment: A Reader in Participation and Development.* London: Zed Books, 1995.

Mink, G. *Welfare's End.* Ithaca, N.Y.: Cornell University Press, 1998.

Minkler, M. "Introduction and Overview." In M. Minkler (ed.), *Community Organizing and Community Building for Health.* New Brunswick, N.J.: Rutgers University Press, 2002.

Minkler, M., and Wallerstein, N. "Improving Health Through Community Organization and Community Building: A Health Education Perspective." In M. Minkler (ed.), *Community Organizing and Community Building for Health.* New Brunswick, N.J.: Rutgers University Press, 2002.

Mintz, S. *Sweetness and Power: The Place of Sugar in Modern History.* New York: Viking Press, 1985.

Murty, S. A., and others. "Physical and Emotional Partner Abuse Reported by Men and Women in a Rural Community." *American Journal of Public Health,* 2000, *93,* 1073–1075.

Nair, C., Karim, R. and Nyers, C. "Health Care and Health Status: A Canadian–United States Statistical Comparison." *Health Reports*, 1992, *4*, 175–182.

National Center for Complementary and Alternative Medicine. "The Use of Complementary and Alternative Medicine by the American Public." *NCCAM Newsletter*, Summer 2003, pp. 1–9.

National Center for Health Statistics. *Health, United States, 2001: Urban and Rural Health Chartbook*. Hyattsville, Md.: National Center for Health Statistics, 2001.

National Center for Health Statistics. *Health United States, 2002*. Hyattsville, Md.: National Center for Health Statistics, 2002.

National Center for Health Statistics. *Health United States, 2003*. Hyattsville, Md.: National Center for Health Statistics, 2003.

New York City Department of City Planning. *The Newest New Yorkers, 1990–1994*. New York: New York City Department of City Planning, 1996.

Nolan, P. A. "Primary Prevention with the Poor: Structural Conflicts Between the Health and Welfare Systems." In M. J. Holosko and M. D. Feit (eds.), *Health and Poverty*. Binghamton, N.Y.: Haworth Press, 1997.

Northridge, M., and Shepard, P. "Environmental Racism and Public Health." *American Journal of Public Health*, 1997, *87*, 730–732.

Norton, B. L., and others. "Community Capacity: Concept, Theory, and Methods." In R. J. Di Clemente, R. A. Crosby, and M. C. Kegler (eds.), *Emerging Theories in Health Promotion Practice and Research*. San Francisco: Jossey-Bass, 2002.

O'Gorman, F. "Brazilian Community Development: Changes and Challenges." In G. Craig and M. Mayo (eds.), *Community Empowerment: A Reader in Participation and Development*. London: Zed Books, 1995.

Pappas, G. "Editorial." *American Journal of Public Health*, 1994, *84*, 892–893.

Paul, B. D. *Health, Culture, and Community: Case Studies of Public Reactions to Health Programs*. New York: Russell Sage Foundation, 1955.

Payer, L. *Medicine and Culture: Varieties of Treatment in the United States, England, West Germany, and France*. New York: Henry Holt, 1988.

Rawaf, S., and Bahl, V. *Assessing Health Needs of People from Minority Ethnic Groups*. London: Royal College of Physicians, Faculty of Public Health Medicine, 1998.

Read, M. *Culture, Health, and Disease: Social and Cultural Influences on Health Programs in Developing Countries*. Philadelphia: Lippincott, 1966.

Riese, H. *Heal the Hurt Child*. Chicago: University of Chicago Press, 1962.

Rivera, F. G., and Erlich, J. L. "A Time of Fear, a Time of Hope." In F. G. Rivera and J. L. Erlich (eds.), *Community Organizing in a Diverse Society*. Boston: Allyn & Bacon, 1998.

Root, J., and Stableford, S. "Easy-to-Read Consumer Communications: A Missing Link in Medicaid Management Care." *Journal of Health Politics, Policy and Law,* 1999, *24,* 1–26.

Rosen, G. "The Community and the Health Officer: A Working Team." *American Journal of Public Health,* 1954, *44,* 14–16.

Rosenthal, B. "How to Build Effective Multicultural Coalitions: Inclusivity Checklist." In M. Minkler (ed.), *Community Organizing and Community Building for Health.* New Brunswick, N.J.: Rutgers University Press, 2002.

Rubin, H. J. "Economic Partnering with the Poor: Why Local Governments Should Work with Community-Based Development Organizations to Promote Economic Development." *International Journal of Public Administration,* 2000, *23,* 1697–1701.

Rubin, H. J., and Rubin, I. S. *Community Organizing and Development.* (2nd ed.) Boston: Allyn & Bacon, 2001.

Saleeby, H. J. "Culture, Theory, and Narrative: The Intersection of Meanings in Practice." *Social Work,* 1994, *39,* 351–359.

Saunders, L. *Cultural Difference and Medical Care: The Case of the Spanish-Speaking People of the Southwest.* New York: Russell Sage Foundation, 1954.

Seifert, K. L., and Hoffnung, R. J. *Child and Adolescent Development.* (3rd ed.) Boston: Houghton Mifflin, 1994.

Shanahan, P., and Ward, J. "The University and Empowerment: The European Union, University Adult Education and Community Economic Development with 'Excluded Groups.'" In G. Craig and M. Mayo (eds.), *Community Empowerment: A Reader in Participation and Development.* London: Zed Books, 1995.

Sidel, R. *Women and Children Last: The Plight of Poor Women in Affluent America.* New York: Penguin Books, 1986.

Singh, G. K., and Yu, S. M. "Infant Mortality in the United States: Trends, Differentials, and Projections, 1950 through 2010." *American Journal of Public Health,* 1995, *85,* 957–964.

Stafford, W. W. *Black Civil Society and the Black Family in New York City: A Struggle for Inclusion in Decision Making.* New York: Black Family Task Force, Manhattan Borough President's Office, 1997.

Starr, P. *The Social Transformation of American Medicine: The Rise of a Sovereign Profession and the Making of a Vast Industry.* New York: Basic Books, 1982.

Thomas, S. B., and Quinn, S. C. "The Tuskegee Syphilis Study, 1932–1972: Implications for HIV Education and AIDS Risk Programs in the Black Community." *American Journal of Public Health,* 1991, *91,* 1498–1505.

Thorpe, K. E., and Knickman, J. R. "Financing for Health Care." In A. R. Kovner and S. Jonas (eds.), *Health Care Delivery in the United States.* (7th ed.) New York: Springer, 2002.

U.S. Census Bureau. *Poverty in the United States, 2001.* Washington, D.C.: Government Printing Office, 2001.

U.S. Department of Health and Human Services. *Report of the Secretary's Task Force on Black and Minority Health.* Washington, D.C.: Government Printing Office, 1985.

Vega, W. A., Sribney, W. M., and Achara-Abrahams, I. "Co-Occurring Alcohol, Drug, and Other Psychiatric Disorders Among Mexican-Origin People in the United States." *American Journal of Public Health,* 2003, *93,* 1057–1064.

Walzer, M. *What It Means to Be an American: Essays on the American Experience.* New York: Marsilio, 1992.

Wandersman, A., Goodman, R. M., and Butterfoss, F. D. "Understanding Coalitions and How They Operate: An 'Open Systems' Organizational Framework." In M. Minkler (ed.), *Community Organizing and Community Building for Health.* New Brunswick, N.J.: Rutgers University Press, 2002.

Weinberg, D. H. *Press Briefing on 2001 Income and Poverty Estimates.* Washington, D.C.: U.S. Census Bureau, 2002.

Williams, D. R. "The Monitoring of Racial/Ethnic Status in the USA: Data Quality Issues." *Ethnicity and Health,* 1999, *4,* 121–137.

Wilson, M., and Daly, M. "Life Expectancy, Economic Inequality, Homicide, and Reproductive Timing in Chicago Neighborhoods." In I. Kawachi, B. P. Kennedy, and R. G. Wilkinson (eds.), *The Society and Population Health Reader: Income Inequality and Health.* New York: New Press, 1999.

World Health Organization. "Ottawa Charter for Health Promotion." *Canadian Journal of Public Health,* 1986, 77, 425–430.

Zambrana, R. E., Dorrington, C., and Bell, S. A. "Mexican Women in Higher Education: A Comparative Study." *Race, Gender, and Class,* 1997, *4,* 127–149.

Zimmerman, R. "Social Equity and Environmental Risk." *Risk Analysis,* 1993, *13,* 649–666.

Community-Based Health Organizations: Essential Functions and Ongoing Challenges

The two chapters in Part Two address the functions and uses of community-based health organizations.

Chapter Three reports on findings from data collected from more than sixty CBHOs across the United States. The focus is on best practices and lessons learned. A typology of the various models of service delivery used by CBHOs in the study to encourage utilization of services and the various characteristics of those models are included.

Chapter Four presents a case study that draws on the twenty years of experience of a local New York City community-based organization, the Caribbean Women's Health Association, Inc. It defines the Health Keepers Model and examines the theoretical approaches on which the model rests. It explains how such a model, though requiring more complex systems and relationships, is capable of significant community penetration, involvement, and development. It also describes why this model is effective when employed by small, local entities. The chapter concludes with some possible new approaches

CBHOs could consider in order to strengthen their capacity to adjust to the broader forces of politics, economics, cultural trends, immigration, and community needs.

Highlighted throughout both chapters are the essential roles that community-based health organizations play in the spectrum of health care delivery and the challenges they face in building and sustaining their infrastructure.

Chapter Three

CBHOs:
A Research Report

Marcia Bayne Smith
Sally Guttmacher

The study discussed in this chapter is an early contribution to what we project will be years of continuous research on community health in general and on community-based health organizations (CBHOs) in particular, not just in the United States but around the world. This projection rests on the recent but growing literature on community health (McKenzie, Pinger, and Kotecki, 2002; Reagan and Brookins-Fisher, 2002) and on community-focused health care (Rohde and Wyon, 2002; Wurzbach, 2002).

Therefore, this study was undertaken with the primary intent of focusing attention on CBHOs as a critical format for the delivery of community health services that has not yet been carefully examined. We hope that health care practitioners and researchers will want to build and improve on this groundwork study. Areas for further work include efforts to increase the sample size and delve more deeply into the issues raised here. Consequently, the study discussed in this chapter should be approached as a prelude to the work that still lies ahead for all of us.

As we go forward, research must include the role of CBHOs in advancing the work of community organizing and building social

The authors wish to thank Savannah Shyne, MPH, for her assistance with this research.

capital, cohesion, civil society, and empowerment as described in the chapters in Part One. These processes of change, from organizing to empowerment, do not occur in some poor communities. As a result, they are less likely to negotiate equal partnerships that can contribute to improving community health. This chapter draws on the theoretical paradigms presented in Chapter Two to help explain the role of CBHOs in community change and improving community health.

Learning Objectives

- Although CBHOs share many similarities, there are large differences among them in terms of structure, mission, and internal and external operations.
- The budgets, staffing, and numbers of clients seen vary greatly among CBHOs.
- All of the CBHOs in our sample with budgets over $20 million per year were started prior to 1988, and more than half of these were started prior to 1971.
- The origins of CBHOs may differ, although they seem to fall into a pattern.
- CBHOs could use media more effectively.
- CBHOs must have a mission statement that provides a guide for all of the organization's activities and programs.
- All of the organizations in this study established within the past ten years have budgets under $5 million.
- The board of directors of an organization commonly sets the organization's policy and is the public face of the organization. It gives the organization greater legitimacy in the eyes of the outside world.
- The organizational structure of a CBHO should be laid out in its important documents, which include the table of organization, constitution and by-laws, strategic plan, and fund development plan.

Background of the CBHO Study

CBHOs such as those that participated in this study were defined in Chapter One as entities established by or in partnership with community-based groups to deliver health, mental health, or health-related social and support services to that community. Most of the CBHOs in this study are not-for-profit entities, including federally funded 330 community health centers (CHCs).

There is an extensive literature on the nonprofit sector (Abramson and Salamon, 1986; Wolf, 1999) and its social service agencies in general (Alexander, 1999; Alexander, Nank, and Stivers, 1999), community organizing specifically (Halpern, 1995; Brager, Specht, and Torczyner, 1987), and community-based organizations in particular (Halpern, 1995). The literature concentrates on CHCs that are part of the federal 330 system (Bureau of Primary Health Care, 1996). During the 1990s, much of this literature on nonprofits focused on the problems faced by a majority of CHCs, such as inherent difficulties in conducting outcome evaluation of services provided by community clinics (Wells and Conviser, 1998), the capacity of CHCs to transition into the managed care mode of capitated care and fixed budgets (Nadel, 1995), and their continued roles as nonprofits in a managed care system (Schlesinger, Gray, and Bradley, 1996) and as providers of comprehensive primary care services to the underserved (Schauffler and Wolin, 1996). However, not much has been documented about the internal or external operations of CBHOs that deliver health or health-related social and support services.

Research on CBHOs as not-for-profit entities has been mindful of the care that CBHOs must take to assess their current operations, engage in strategic planning, and carefully prepare for changes to come (Salamon, 1996; Light, 2000). Some of the literature predicted changes that could occur over time. For example, one study on CBHOs indicated that one of the key staffing categories used in these organizations, community health workers, has now become an integral occupation in the health care workforce (Witmer and others, 1995).

Other studies have pointed to the important bridge that some community organizations have become in relaying community health needs to health care providers (Irigoyen and Findley, 1998). However, very few studies have examined the internal and external operations of CBHOs with the aim of gaining a better understanding of them. As CBHOs proliferate, form partnerships, and become integral components of the health services system, there is a need to know more about them. Some of the areas of interest include how they emerged, their missions, how they currently function, and how they manage their relationships to multiple levels of stakeholders in the community they serve in a changing political and economic climate. An equally important area of interest is how they maintain organizational stability while adapting to change.

Study Rationale

This dearth of information points to the need to begin gathering information on CBHOs. More information is necessary to determine how involved they are with organizing and building their internal operations as well as developing their external relationships to the community they serve and to the broader community, including other community health organizations and institutions. The study discussed in this chapter was designed to provide empirical data on CBHOs about their purpose, as stated in their mission statements; the clients they serve; their staffing, structure, and governance; programs and services offered; their relationship with their external environment, especially with clients; and efforts to engage in planning and evaluation.

Aims of the Study

One of our primary aims was to investigate how our theoretical understanding of CBHOs helps explain differences or similarities in their current structure, mission, past and future challenges, and funding sources. The question that seems most pressing for the future of such organizations is, What attributes of a CBHO help maintain organizational stability and growth over time? It is therefore essential to understand how CBHOs function internally, particularly in their relationship with clients and the community. This relationship includes client input into internal programming, which, from a political economy approach, with its emphasis on balancing inequality, is more in keeping with "power with" and "power to" than "power over" (Minkler, 2002, p. 8). Therefore, client input is essentially an indication of the power that community members have in determining the organization's goals and how the organization functions to meet them. In addition, we need to understand the role that CBHOs play in supporting other community social structures, which entails investigating the external relationships and partnerships CBHOs have been able to develop at various levels of their community.

Methodology

Sixty-five CBHOs in eighteen states plus the District of Columbia, with annual budgets ranging from under $1 million to over $20 million, were studied in 2003 to evaluate their internal and external operations. These organizations typified the scope of CBHOs: some had been in existence for a century or more and some for only a dozen years. All of the organizations that responded answered a questionnaire sent to them by fax or electronic mail, with the exception of two sites that requested the survey be mailed to them. Six sites were selected from the sample to participate in case studies that included in-depth interviews with the chief executive officer or executive director.

The clients served by the sixty-five CBHOs in the sample represent the full gamut of racial, ethnic, and cultural groups in the United States. However, the unit of analysis was the CBHO, not individual clients. Therefore, the study did not require approval of Institutional Review Board's Committees for the Protection of Human Subjects at any of the institutions or affiliations.

Study Design

This was a cross-sectional study designed to collect onetime data on relevant variables in two different formats. An in-depth interview was conducted with six CBHOs, using an unstructured questionnaire that was administered by an interviewer either in person or by telephone with someone in an administrative capacity. In addition, a self-administered survey was sent electronically or through the mail. Data collected from both methodologies were used in the following analysis.

Sampling

A combined list of CBHOs was assembled from the Web sites of the Bureau of Primary Health Care (BPHC) and the United Way. The BPHC is part of the Health Resources and Services Administration (HRSA), which itself is part of the U.S. Department of Health and Human Services. The BPHC has a database of community-based free or low-cost primary care services, all of which receive some funding from the HRSA-BPHC program described in Chapter One.

The HRSA-BPHC funding is a federal grant program under section 330 of the Public Health Services Act designed to provide primary and preventive health care services in medically underserved areas throughout the United States and its territories. United Way is a national membership organization that serves primarily as a conduit for private and philanthropic donations that United Way disburses to local organizational members (CBOs and CBHOs). In addition, United Way provides members with technical assistance in capacity building.

A random sample of five hundred CBHOs was drawn from this combined list. Telephone calls were made to identify the manager or site director as well as the appropriate person in the agency to complete the questionnaire. Follow-up calls were made following dispatch of the questionnaires and accompanying cover letters; questionnaires that had been lost in transit were replaced.

Of the five hundred questionnaires distributed, sixty-five usable responses were received, a return rate of 13 percent. In addition to the survey, six unstructured interviews were carried out with CBHO directors by members of the project staff. Although this response rate of 13 percent might be deemed as low by most typical survey standards (Lynn, Beerten, Laiho, and Martin, 2001), three particular issues must be considered here. First, we did not employ any of the many strategies that could be used to boost survey response rate, as our emphasis was not necessarily on obtaining the largest possible universe *(N)* for this study. Our focus was on getting to know as much as we could from a representative sample of CBHOs about how these organizations operated internally and externally in their efforts to improve community health.

Second, the goal was less on rigorous in-depth analyses and more on examining CBHOs as a health service delivery medium and on discovering if they were legitimate entities in which serious internal efforts were undertaken to substantively involve community members in developing and delivering health services. Finally, we were also interested in obtaining a close-up look at the external operations of CBHOs—their connections to their external environment, including community-based organizations, elected officials, and other stakeholders. These relationships are considered critical if CBHOs are to serve as catalysts for building and empowering communities to advocate for improved health. Therefore, we established criteria for inclusion in the study and conducted the study on those respondents that were eligible.

Criteria

The size of the universe of CBHOs in the United States is unknown in part because of the inherent instability of this particular type of organization within the general CBO-nonprofit genre. New CBHOs are constantly founded while others are closing down. Nevertheless, there are specific characteristics that encompass the essential elements of CBHOs. Therefore, our goal was to obtain a sample that would be representative of this population by developing the following criteria from which the final sample was selected:

1. The CBHO must have a community base. If the CBHO is partnered or is affiliated with a hospital, medical center, or university, it operates nevertheless as an autonomous entity.
2. The CBHO must have its own mission statement.
3. The CBHO must already have or be working on incorporation as a legal entity and obtaining 501(c)(3) federal tax-exempt status.
4. The CBHO must respond by a specific cutoff date or time frame for response, generally four months.

The sixty-five respondents admitted to the study met all four of these criteria.

Sample Size

Commercial and economic surveys customarily tout survey response rates as high as 80 to 90 percent. However, current research suggests that those rates have dropped precipitously in recent years (Sheehan and McMillan, 1999). The decreased response to e-mailed surveys appears to be following a general pattern of declining survey response rates in general in the United States. This trend has been attributed to a variety of causes, which are addressed in the discussion section of this chapter. Cognizant of the fact that the response rate to mailed (paper and electronic) survey questionnaires has shown a continuous decrease, we established the goal of achieving a return rate of at least 10 percent. Our 13 percent rate of useful responses was therefore considered successful.

Survey Development and Field Testing

An earlier version of the survey instrument was developed for use as part of a prior study (Bayne Smith, 1996). That instrument was revised for use in this study, based on input from colleagues at Queens College. Subsequently, each of the authors made additional revisions that led to the final instrument. The final instrument was then piloted with two CBHOs in the New York City area, two in the Washington, D.C., area, and one in San Francisco. During the pilot study, the instrument was rated favorably with respect to user friendliness, ease of reading, clarity of questions, and consistency.

Qualitative data from in-depth interviews were also collected to flesh out some of the questionnaire data. These interviews were guided by a set of questions designed to facilitate the discussion and conducted with people who had been intimately connected with the development and progress of six CBHOs from their inception. Three of these were from the New York metropolitan area and the others were from Miami, Washington, and New Orleans. The discussion in this chapter weaves the two types of data together to give a clear picture of the development of such organizations.

Analysis

The analysis conducted on this database was essentially descriptive. In some instances, we looked for differences according to the size of the organization using the yearly organizational budget as the measure of size. The rationale for this kind of comparison is provided by our hypotheses, which are that budget size is closely associated with having a well-thought-out internal structure and that budgets will increase rather than decrease when CBHOs have strong relationships with their external environment. Correlations were run between thirty-five key variables in an effort to determine what relationships existed, if any, between variables.

Results

Exhibit 3.1 lists the locations of the CBHOs participating in this study. Their characteristics are profiled in Table 3.1.

For the purposes of this study, organizations with budgets under $5 million are referred to as small, those with budgets between

Exhibit 3.1. Locations of Participating CBHOs.

California: Concord, Oakland, San Diego	Missouri: Saint Louis
Colorado: Denver	New Jersey: Hackensack
District of Columbia: Washington	New York: New York City (Brooklyn, Manhattan)
Florida: Miami	Pennsylvania: Philadelphia
Georgia: Atlanta	Rhode Island: Providence
Iowa: Des Moines	Texas: San Antonio
Kentucky: Louisville	Virginia: Richmond
Louisiana: New Orleans	Washington: Seattle
Maryland: Baltimore	Wisconsin: Milwaukee
Massachusetts: Boston	

$5 and $20 million are designated as medium, and those with budgets over $20 million are deemed large.

Internal Operations of CBHOs

The results reported here describe primarily how CBHOs function internally. Internal functioning includes mission statements, organizational structure, board, personnel, organizational planning, client profile, services provided, finances and funding, and past and future challenges.

The Mission of CBHOs

All participating CBHOs in the sample indicated that they did have a mission statement, although not all included it with their returned surveys. Of the fifty-one organizations that submitted mission statements, most reported revising the statement within the past three years, and almost all report that their activities are guided by their mission statement.

A lengthy description of mission statements is provided by Below, Morrisey, and Acomb (1987). Put most simply, the mission statement is a succinct statement that encapsulates the purpose of the organization, its goals, and the population and geographical area to be served. It is often displayed in a prominent place that is readily visible upon entering the organization.

Table 3.1. Characteristics of Participating CBHOs.

Variable	Frequency	Percentage	Cumulative Percentage
Date of Founding			
1883–1970	11	17.7	17.7
1971–1980	20	32.3	50.0
1981–1990	19	30.6	80.6
1991–2003	12	19.4	90.0
3 missing responses		100.0	
Size of Staff			
1–25	18	28.6	28.6
26–100	20	31.7	60.3
>100	25	39.0	99.3
3 missing responses		100.0	
Clients Served			
27–1000	39	60.0	60.0
1,000–40,000	19	25.0	85.0
40,000–100,000	5	9.0	94.0
2 missing responses		100.0	
Budget			
$1,000,000	9	17.0	17.0
$1,000,000–$4,999,000	17	34.0	50.9
$5,000,000–$20,000,000	15	28.3	79.2
$20,000,000	11	20.8	99.0
12 missing responses		100.0	

Many of the mission statements we received were specific to the provision of health care services to populations in a caring manner, and most mention that their services are culturally sensitive. Here is an example:

The ABC Neighborhood Health Center's mission is to provide comprehensive health care to individuals and families who have difficulty accessing care, respond with sensitivity to the needs of our diverse patients, and advocate and work with others to improve the overall health status of the communities we serve.

Other CBHOs surveyed were broader in their definition of health, incorporating into their mission statement the goals of "advocacy for equity" or "community empowerment." In doing so, they made the activities required to achieve those goals intrinsic components in the provision of services for all of the underserved. For example:

To improve the wellness of the New Orleans community by providing culturally competent, comprehensive health care services and training and by participating in a community-directed, antiracist process of self-determination.

Some mission statements included the provision of shelter or the elimination of homelessness as part of their mission, and some have as their mission the achievement of changes in social policy as well as delivery of care:

The ABC Agency of New York City works to ameliorate the devastating effects of homelessness by ensuring a wide array of high-quality support services to people experiencing homelessness and by helping bring about substantial improvements in policies and programs affecting homeless people. ABC places at the core of all our work the ultimate goal of eliminating homelessness within our city and country.

Many organizations, however, define their missions in more specific terms. For example, some specify providing health and wellness care, health education, or referral services for specific types of health problems such as psychiatric illness or substance abuse:

XYZ is a nonprofit psychiatric rehabilitation organization that ensures a supportive community for adults with long-term psychiatric disabilities so that they can develop living, learning, working, and social skills and access the resources needed to lead and sustain successful and satisfying lives.

Some mission statements include the names of specific ethnic groups, such as Haitians, Hispanics, or Asians. For example:

To serve and advocate for the immigrant and refugee Asian community regarding its health rights and to ensure access to health care services regardless of income, insurance status, language, or culture.

> The QRS Community Health Center is a community-based organization com-
> mitted to providing quality, comprehensive health and human services to
> diverse communities, specializing in service to Hispanic community residents.

All say that they are sensitive to community and cultural diversity, although a few harked back to the days of clinics founded by
Christian missionaries with specifically Christian faith-based mission statements such as this:

> To proclaim and demonstrate the Gospel of Jesus Christ, meeting the spiritual,
> physical, and emotional needs of men, women, and children who are home-
> less and in need of assistance.

The significance of the mission statement cannot be too strongly
stated or reiterated too often. It is the critical first step that provides
clear purpose, intention, and direction for the organization. The examples cited here show that it must be approached and formulated
with great care and precision.

Development of CBHOs

Some CBHOs are started as an individual or group response to a
perceived or expressed need. Others are set up in response to funding that is made available to tackle a specific health or social issue.
Their beginnings must be viewed in their historical context, that is,
in terms of the expressed concerns of society at a particular time.
Some are founded by groups of professionals who are concerned
about a particular at risk group or community:

> It was a time when there was a lot of interest. Usually programs get developed
> "after the fact" of the need or because that program will respond to the "prob-
> lem of the month." But our organization began not to just go after funding for
> pregnancy. We were trying to educate those who fund to think more holisti-
> cally. It was like wildfire. . . . In the first few weeks, there was a hundred young
> people a night streaming in. It was really an incredible time and also an op-
> portunity for this interdisciplinary group of professionals not just to provide
> services to young people that were there but also to be able, slowly over time,
> to change systems and how they treated young people.

Others are started by individuals responding to a perceived or expressed need in the community:

> She set up a clinic in the lobby of that apartment building, and in little more
> than a year, it had grown so much that they had to move into a two-bedroom

apartment. This was 1976, and within a year after that, we obtained a three-year grant from the Kellogg Foundation for $500,000 to set up a new Holistic Health Services center. A couple of years later, the Holistic part of the name was dropped because of misinterpretations of that word, but the commitment to comprehensive heath services remained. It became incorporated May 1, 1979, and a year later moved into its current space. At first there were just a couple of doctors, but slowly more doctors and services, such as mental health and addiction counseling services, have been added. The expansion has also been in terms of hours of operation as well as in terms of partnership.

Finally, some CBHOs first develop as part of other organizations and eventually split off as independent entities:

We were based at a host agency. We grew and got federal money and then Ryan White money and became almost bigger than our host organization. We explored a number of options, thinking that we would get adopted by some organization. We decided to separately incorporate and in January 1993 really became independent. After this, all grants for us that had previously come through our host came to us directly.

I was told that there was this pot of money that the legislature had to spend and it must be used for outreach to hard-to-reach populations. It was NIH money, and they never provide money for services, as their only interest is research. I immediately thought, I have got to use this money for homeless youth services. This was absolutely perfect. So I partnered with the local AIDS task force (NOAIDS) to work with and wrote the proposal. At any rate, I ended up with an adolescent drop-in center. The first place we got was a small room with the ceiling falling in on us, where we could see adolescents twice a week for medical care.

Evident throughout all of these examples are collaborative efforts among professionals, funding agencies, and the clients being served, as well as the need for interorganizational support whereby one organization provides space to or hosts another. This level of collaboration and interdisciplinarity is needed not only at startup but also, as we shall see, for the ongoing sustainability of CBHOs.

The Structure of CBHOs

About half of the CBHOs surveyed had budgets of less than $5 million a year, and one-fifth had budgets over $20 million. The organizations with the larger budgets had more full-time and part-time staff. The large organizations offered a wider range of services. All but one of the large CBHOs provided health services, and the majority offered mental health services as well. Over half (55 percent) of the organizations with budgets over $20 million included services related to housing. Employment training and child welfare services were much more typical of services provided by smaller organizations.

Although most of the respondents in the sample were affiliated with other organizations, the very large CBHOs in our sample were more likely to report getting funds from their affiliates. They were also more likely to serve as satellite clinics and as a host site for interns.

To maintain stability over time and to support their ability to grow, CBHOs must have a formal structure. Having a constitution and by-laws, an executive director, a functioning board of directors, and a description of the organizational hierarchy is evidence of structure. In fact, most (80 percent) of the sixty-five organizations that responded have a constitution and by-laws. Even more (90 percent) have a board of directors and a full-time executive director. Only two had volunteer executive directors.

The Board

The board of directors of an organization commonly sets the organization's policy and is the public face of the organization. It gives the organization legitimacy in the eyes of the outside world. Indeed, the board of directors of a nonprofit organization represents a vital link for that organization to its external environment. All but two of the CBHOs surveyed have a board of directors, and these two organizations had very small budgets of less than $1 million per year. Frequently, boards evolve after the founding of the organization once the mission of the organization becomes clearer, as exemplified by one interviewee:

> The core people turned into the board of directors (probably around 1975), as by that time it was clear that we were really building an organization and pushing for nonprofit status. This group provided the leadership for each of the core areas.

The makeup of the board informs us about the board's strengths and its ability to do outreach and communicate with the community, to evaluate the success of reaching those they intend to serve, and to represent the organization in the broader external environment and presumably help with the perception of legitimacy within a community. The CBHOs surveyed reported the following board composition:

88 percent had board members from the racial and ethnic groups served.

72 percent had board members who were consumers of services.

69 percent had board members who were professional providers.

83 percent had board members who were community leaders.

80 percent had board members with access to resources.

To further tease out information regarding access to resources, respondents were asked about the availability of board members in various critical resource areas. They reported the following:

67 percent had board members involved in public relations.

64 percent had board members involved in fundraising.

52 percent had board members with fundraising skills and expertise.

20 percent had board members with grant-writing skills.

Note that almost all (88 percent) of the boards of directors of the organizations surveyed include representatives of the ethnic groups served. This is important in terms of keeping the organization accountable in meeting the needs of clients and the various groups in the local community. A mix of board members was not uncommon among those surveyed, as board members are also relied on to help connect CBHOs to those segments of the larger community among whom significant funds can be raised. CBHOs are often required to engage in producing matching funds and in other kinds of fundraising by both public and private funding sources.

Except for the very small CBHOs, over two-thirds of the medium- to large-size organizations have consumers of the services sitting on the board whose special contribution would be to give the board feedback related to problems with service delivery. The importance of having consumers on the board was expressed by one of our interviewees:

> The board has a patient majority and also reflects the demographics of the population served. The board has input into all services, creates a survey, and

administers it to about 20 percent of patients annually to obtain their input about what they like, what is working, what they do not like or is not working, and what they would like to see.

The specific activity of the board in relation to the CBHO varies. On the whole, boards are not involved in the day-to-day management of the organization. Most boards are involved in making or approving the policies of the organization, and most have financial oversight responsibilities. A very important function of the board is to see that the organization remains stable and well resourced. The larger organizations were more likely to report board members engaged in this type of activity. Over two-thirds of the organizations, regardless of size, reported that board members are involved in fundraising, and all of the larger budgeted CBHOs and most of the smaller ones in our sample had board members with financial skills. Most of the larger CBHOs reported board members with legal skills as well. This was slightly less likely in the smaller organizations. Slightly more than two-thirds have a member with legal expertise and experience in public relations. Two-fifths (39 percent) of the CBHOs report that their board is involved in preparing the annual budget, and most (86 percent) indicate that the board reviews financial reports.

Personnel Liability

The personnel in most of the CBHOs surveyed were covered by general liability insurance as well as professional liability insurance. However, one-third of the smaller CBHOs did not have liability insurance, which includes medical insurance, leaving the personnel vulnerable to major financial burdens if they become ill and do not have other types of third-party insurance. Lack of such coverage might indicate a potential lack of stability in retaining personnel. In the larger organizations, the officers and directors were covered by liability insurance, whereas less than half of very small CBHOs with budgets under $1 million provide such coverage for their directors.

Organizational Planning

Most of the CBHOs indicated having a well-developed organizational structure, as reflected by the planning documents they indicated that were maintained on file. Three-quarters have a strategic or long-range plan on file, and almost two-thirds (65 percent) have an operational or short-term plan filed. Almost all of the larger organizations have a quality assurance plan in place to ascertain the quality of the services they provide, whereas this was true of only two-fifths of the small to medium-size organizations with budgets below $5 million. Almost all the CBHOs' files included job descriptions, an employee's handbook, and staff evaluations. Most organizations produce an annual report of board activities, including the annual budget, which is usually prepared by a financial officer or the executive director.

Client Profile

Table 3.2 presents a profile of the clients served by the participating CBHOs. Three key pieces of information stand out:

- Practically all the organizations surveyed (93 percent) are serving low-income populations, and 85 percent of all CBHOs in this study are serving people who are uninsured, many of whom must pay out of pocket because they lack insurance. This raises a serious question: While all CBHOs face similar demographic shifts, how are the small to medium-size organizations dealing with this? In other words, how are they staying alive if they are not being adequately reimbursed for their services?
- More than two-thirds (68 percent) are serving large immigrant populations.
- Half of all the organizations in this study indicated that they now serve a population that is less than 10 percent white. Some serve populations that are more than 75 percent black, Asian, or Hispanic. This type of patient mix indicates that CBHOs serve a client base that consists of largely poor, uninsured racial and ethnic minorities. This population is likely to have more health problems and less access to care at the larger health care institutions, thus making CBHOs a vital link in the nation's health system.

Services Provided

The CBHOs surveyed are providing the following services:

Health services (86 percent)

Mental health services, including chemical dependency treatment programs (72 percent)

Social work services (88 percent)

Table 3.2. Profile of Clients Served.

Variable	Frequency	Percentage
Clients from Geographical Target Areas		
Local neighborhood	47	72
Borough or county	28	43
City or municipality	46	71
Statewide	12	19
National	5	8
Client Demographics		
Youths to age 19 years	56	86
Adults	57	88
Seniors	47	72
Males	56	86
Females	58	89
Low-income	61	93
Uninsured	55	85
Immigrants	44	68
Racial groups:		
< 10% white	31	49
> 75% Asian	2	3
> 75% Hispanic	6	10
> 75% black	14	22
Numbers Served Annually		
27–1,000	15	25
1,001–10,000	19	30.8
10,001–40,000	20	29.2
40,001–100,000	5	7.7
Missing	6	9.2
Total	65	100.0
Change in Number of Clients in Past Two Years		
Decrease	6	9.2
No change	12	18.5
Increased	44	71.0
Missing	3	99.0
Total	65	100.0

Housing (40 percent)

Immigration services (12 percent)

Employment or job training (29 percent)

Child welfare (11 percent)

After-school programs for children and adolescents (22 percent)

And these services are provided in the following manner:

Information and referrals (80 percent)

Case management (89 percent)

Advocacy (71 percent)

Counseling (75 percent)

Clinical services through primary and specialty care clinics that provide primary care, mental health, dental, and substance abuse and family planning services (74 percent)

Finances and Funding

Over three-quarters of the CBHOs surveyed claim to have board members with access to resources. Such access is important for fundraising. In 69 percent of the CBHOs, the manager or executive director is in charge of locating funds for the organization, and most (83 percent) have individual staff members (executive director, manager, or management team) who is responsible for writing grant proposals. Only nine (14 percent) reported that they hired an independent consultant to write their grants, whereas four organizations reported having a development director whose job included writing grant proposals.

Expenses are commonly monitored by the chief financial officer or the executive director, and in most organizations surveyed (83 percent), financial reports are submitted by them on a monthly basis. The smaller organizations were less likely to have their financial and policy procedures on file, but almost all (97 percent) report being audited annually. Nearly as many of the CBHOs surveyed (94 percent) carry liability insurance.

Most nongovernmental organizations must have plans for maintaining current funding and procuring future funding. Thus it is surprising that only a few of the organizations (11 percent) had independent consultants responsible for locating outside funding and only five organizations had a development director. Over three-quarters of the larger organizations had a plan for the development of funds; however, such a plan was less common in the smaller organizations, where over one-third had none. For those who did, these plans included grant writing (63 percent), planning special events (52 percent) or solicitation campaigns (43 percent), getting an endowment (31 percent) or individual donations (54 percent), asking for employee donations (25 percent), or increasing their reliance on fee-for-service (30 percent). The smallest organizations, with budgets under $1 million, were considerably less likely to consider relying on fee-for-service as a model for future development, nor were they likely to be considering employee contributions or individual donors as a potential source of support.

Ideally, a mix of funding sources is most advantageous for any organization so that if one source dries up, others are available to take up the slack. As one individual told us:

> Our agency has at least a hundred different funding sources now, and it took a lot in the way of creativity to get this kind of funding mix so that we would not be dependent on a particular source (like the government) for funds. There's never been more than 44 to 55 percent dependence on government funds. There was always a balance of corporate and private foundations. This is important because if the wind blows the other way, we don't lose funding.

Clearly, procuring funds is one of the major challenges faced by the organizations we surveyed. Many of them have now moved to rely on fee-for-service from a largely uninsured population and on support for clinic services from private funders, which is a less than perfect solution. As one respondent pointed out:

> The current challenge is that while more patients are uninsured, public insurance only covers $50 to $60 of a visit that costs $100. In addition, medications are not covered, nor are many ancillary services such as lab fees, social services, bilingual translations, or X-rays. As a result, the goal now is to present these new kinds of needs in ways that will help funders understand the amount of things that are not covered and need support.

For CBHOs affiliated with larger institutions like universities, raising funds can present additional difficulties because they are perceived to be well funded by the organizations to which they are attached:

> No one wants to put money into this health center for teens . . . because it belongs to someone else [the university].

Because fundraising is so important and difficult, CBHOs need to devote time to educating funders so that they can understand the need for funds for certain services:

> But that's why our agency was started—not to just go after funding about pregnancy, for example. We were trying to educate those who fund to think more holistically.

Past, Current, and Future Challenges

Most of the organizations interviewed desire to expand their services in the hope of increasing their access to resources. It appears from the interview data that their current challenges in this respect have not changed much since the time of founding. Finding the funds to meet the expanding needs of the organization seems to be the major ongoing challenge. Finding adequate facilities for program activities is mentioned as a challenge by about half of the CBHOs surveyed:

> Then as now, the major challenge for the board has been finding sufficient funding to operate programs, expand, and meet the needs of the different groups served. The director of planning and development is constantly looking for new opportunities for expansion and growth of the work.

Working within a larger bureaucracy can also be a challenge for CBHOs, many of which started because local government bureaucracy was unable to meet the needs of their target population:

> It's been a challenge working with the board of education. We wanted to be involved in how education is delivered, but this is difficult because of all the regulations since the education reforms of the 1970s.

Sometimes the challenge is simply working with one's partners, who may have a slightly different philosophical attitude toward dealing with the problem:

> It became so difficult as the first group we worked with wanted the kids to enter into very structured behavior right away and wouldn't buy into the idea that it takes some kids a while to buy into structures. Some of them can't do it immediately.

External Relationships: Organizing and Building Community on Various Levels

In investigating the external relationships and partnerships that CBHOs have developed at various levels in their community, we focused on three components that we consider critical: relationships with the clients served, the use of tools and mechanisms for communicating not only with clients but also with the community at large, and relationships with policymakers. As discussed earlier, clients are the natural constituency base of CBHOs, and it is critical that mechanisms and tools exist for communicating with them. Equally important are elected officials, as many of the CBHOs indicated in their mission statements that advocacy and community empowerment were intrinsic to the provision of services. In that regard, advocacy efforts of CBHOs can be facilitated by the relationships they maintain with elected officials.

Relationship with the Client Base

We have seen that there is great variation in the development paths of CBHOs as well as their explicit missions. Despite this variety, the process that gives birth to CBHOs is almost always a response to a perceived need of some clearly identified group, such as a distinct racial or ethnic population, homeless women, or troubled youth. As part of their development process, most CBHOs engage in some level of community organizing, building, and empowerment, and they do so initially with clients as the natural constituency base of their organizations. One of the ways in which CBHOs organize, build, and empower their community is through the involvement of clients in program planning and design. This type of involvement yields beneficial results in two critical ways. First, clients who provide input into program planning and see their input used to train staff and shape programs and other CBHO activities feel empowered. Second, empowered clients have the potential of becoming the most effective representatives of a CBHO throughout the community.

In addition to the types of services provided by CBHOs discussed earlier, about one-fifth (22 percent) indicated that they are providing after-school programs for children and adolescents. Most (89 percent) were providing case management services for constituent families, which is critically needed in poor and immigrant communities where many residents lack the knowledge or ability to access needed services. Further, as part of the multifaceted approach used by most CBHOs, when asked for "other" services provided, respondents listed a broad range of services that included health education for contraception, child care, and nutrition; family budgeting; leadership building; peer-led health education and counseling; group services; and partnerships with other organizations. These are vital services and programs for children and adults, all of which contribute to community building.

Over two-fifths (42 percent) of the sample said they served distinct ethnic populations for whom services were provided in a linguistically appropriate manner. The most common languages other than English used in the provision of services to clients in our sample were Spanish (84 percent), French (20 percent), Haitian Creole (28 percent), Mandarin (14 percent), and Cantonese (14 percent).

Surprisingly, in response to the question about client population, although two-thirds of the CBHOs reported serving immigrant populations, only 12 percent of the sample provided immigration services for their clients. The significance of specific immigration services for immigrants cannot be overstated. The major concern of every new immigrant is obtaining assistance to legitimize staying in the country if undocumented, and if documented, assistance with processing papers toward family unification. One indication that the service recipients are new immigrants who would greatly benefit from immigration services can be found in the need for services in their own language, which indicates that their arrival is relatively recent and that their level of assimilation has not as yet achieved adequate English-language proficiency.

One of the ways in which CBHOs can determine the need for immigration, linguistic, or other types of services among the clients they serve is to conduct a community needs assessment. This is one of the most effective activities for community organizing and building. The organization conducting the assessment is required to involve multiple levels of the community in providing input into the assessment of both available resources and problems to be addressed. Therefore, conducting a needs assessment provides a unique opportunity to organize and build community around a problem or issue such as health care needs.

The majority (77 percent) of respondents said that they do carry out periodic community needs assessment. Among the fifteen organizations that did not, six indicated that they used some form of client participation method, such as client surveys; patient requests for services; parent, group, and individual meetings; or focus groups, to obtain input and otherwise identify community needs.

Some of the CBHOs who did not carry out periodic community needs assessments indicated that community needs were identified through various other mechanisms, including other local, government, or private reports, statistics, and studies; regional or state office data; state agencies, trade associations, and city agencies; or community organizations with whom they have a partnership.

Although some CBHOs did not conduct formal periodic community needs assessments, almost all of them (97 percent) asked clients for feedback regarding quality of services. The three most often used methods to collect client feedback were survey questionnaires (92 percent), focus groups (61 percent), and word of mouth (25 percent). Several organizations indicated that they used other methods for collecting feedback, such as comment cards in all facilities, a consumer advisory committee, national polls, individual interviews, exit interviews, patient advocates, annual meeting with patients, monthly community meetings, patient advocates, and phone follow-up. As reported earlier, feedback information was then used by respondents to enhance service delivery in the following ways: staff training (86 percent), guiding grants and proposal writing (51 percent), quality management and modifications in service delivery (24 percent), and developing new programs (12 percent.)

Qualitative data from the six in-depth interviews were also useful in providing information on the relationship of the survey respondents to their client base and the community at large. Interviewees indicated that feedback from both clients and the broader community plays a critical role in empowering clients and in the evolution of service programs. One spoke of changes in services as a result of the needs of the organization's teen clients:

> One girl who was a prostitute explained to me that she went to another agency and the staff acted as if she was a baby and needed to be taken care of and she did not like that as she had been taking care of herself since she was twelve. Of course, she was shooting up and doing a lot of other bad things to herself and needed to be taken care of, but that approach did not work for her. That ap-

proach does not work for all kids. She and other kids taught us a lot about how some kids think about prostitution and the need to work with them, to involve them in setting up the necessary structures that they themselves acknowledge that they need but which they must also feel that they had a voice in or contributed to in some way.

Another spoke of intergroup conflicts, community input, and the development of different services for different client groups:

We learned early on of the importance to work with the community and obtain their input as there was a time when our two different sets of clients each had their own name for the health clinic and they competed with each other for resources. We had to work hard to break up the intergroup conflict by doing focus groups and encouraging client participation and input into planning and development for services that best met the needs of the different groups.

Empowered clients are the best source of communication with the larger community. One of the obvious pathways to empowerment is through client participation and input that lead to programmatic changes. Slightly more than three-quarters (77 percent) of the CBHOs in this study sought to enhance client participation through formal, periodic needs assessment, focus groups, and other means of obtaining client input and feedback. In addition, most (97 percent) CBHOs sought feedback from clients regarding quality of services. Even more important, there is evidence that client input and feedback were actually used in revising internal operations, such that more than two-thirds (86 percent) of survey respondents used feedback to enhance service delivery through staff training, and half (51 percent) used client feedback to guide their writing of grants and proposals.

Communicating with the Larger Community

Successful CBHOs engage in organizing and building community with clients. A variety of tools and mechanisms are required to organize effectively and build relationships with both clients and multiple levels of the community as well. Survey respondents were asked if they produced any information and communication tools. More than three-quarters (87 percent) of CBHOs in the study produced brochures, and 81 percent produced an annual report. More than two-thirds of them produced flyers (71 percent) and newsletters (70 percent).

Having established that a majority of CBHOs were indeed producing communication tools, survey participants were asked to indicate if they used these tools to communicate with clients and the general public, and they responded as follows:

Newsletter, brochures, flyers (84 percent)

News conferences (23 percent)

Ethnic print media (28 percent)

Mainstream media, including local TV, newspapers, and radio (53 percent)

Community meetings and programs (73 percent)

Organizational linkages (71 percent)

There were three concerns with these responses. The first is that almost three-quarters (71 percent) said that they communicated with the public through organizational linkages. The expectation was that these organizational linkages were formalized, thereby providing an assured communication and information-sharing pipeline. However, only one-third (34 percent) of the sample have formal linkages with other organizations through a memorandum of understanding.

The second concern is how immigrants, who constitute a large portion of the clients served by survey respondents, are being reached. Two-thirds of those surveyed serve immigrant clients, but only a little more than one-quarter (28 percent) of them use ethnic print media. Mainstream media (newspapers, TV, and radio) can be valuable, depending on location and whether mainstream media in languages other than English exist (as in Miami, where mainstream media are available in both English and Spanish).

The final concern with these responses has to do with one of the major limitations of this study. While it was good to know that these organizations were all doing significant work in terms of communicating with their constituency, what is also important to know is the impact of those communication efforts. However, in the same way that conducting impact analysis is beyond the resources and organizational capability of most small CBHOs, it was also beyond the scope of this study.

Despite these concerns, it certainly must be considered beneficial for immigrant clients not only that a majority of respondents (84 percent) sent out flyers, brochures, and newsletters but also that almost three-quarters (73 percent) of CBHOs reported that they communicated with the public via community meetings and programs. There are multiple benefits to this type of communication. First, a majority of respondents had indicated earlier that they had the capacity to communicate in several languages, which means that clients with poor English-language skills can interact, face to face, with a person who speaks their language. Second, obtaining verbal information in a community meeting or program can be more effective as it allows greater opportunity for interaction, such as asking questions for clarification and providing answers with an opportunity to verify that the correct meaning was conveyed. Third, this kind of interchange is part of a process in which people learn from and teach each other. Fourth, in some communities, written information may be less than effective due to problems with literacy or comprehension.

The ultimate communication capability test in a high-technology and communication-driven world has to do with the ability of CBHOs to access the larger community electronically. The overwhelming majority of respondents (97 percent) indicated that they use computer technology to collect, store, and retrieve data, that their computers were networked, and that they had Internet access.

Advocacy Efforts: Relationships with Policymakers

As noted earlier, some CBHOs' mission statements contained terms such as *advocacy* and *policy change,* which indicates the need to develop relationships with policymakers. Elected officials, as policymakers, are critical to the community-building process as they are important allies in terms of advocating for increased services, securing funding, and obtaining resources to meet identified need. In response to the question, "Does the organization maintain relationships with elected and public officials?" almost all (93 percent) of respondents said yes and specified that they do so in the following ways:

Briefings (46 percent)

Written reports (30 percent)

Regular phone contact (55 percent)

Event planning (57 percent)

In addition, CBHOs reported using a variety of other ways to maintain relationships to elected officials, including informal discussions at meetings, via telephone and newsletters, and through testimony at public hearings. CBHOs make efforts to communicate with elected officials in two separate arenas: as part of CBHO communications with the general public, including elected officials using ethnic print media, and as part of the organizational linkages of CBHOs.

The importance of relationships with elected officials for the organizations surveyed lies in the fact that with the exception of only one, all CBHOs in this study, from the largest to the smallest, receive government funding. Chapter Five takes a more in-depth look at this association between the pursuit of government funds and contracts and the development of solid relationships with elected officials. It should be noted that during the past two years, government funding did increase for a substantial minority of respondent CBHOs (30 percent).

Discussion

Our desire to better understand CBHOs stems from the unique contribution that they are in a position to make to community organizing, building, and empowerment. At the start of this research project, there were many questions for which we were seeking answers. Did our research address those questions? An initial concern has to do with the usefulness of the theoretical understandings of CBHOs for explaining differences and similarities in their current structure, mission, funding sources, and past and future challenges.

Using the political economy perspective, the data on mission statements suggest that CBHOs and other community-based organizations emerge because of the unequal distribution of goods in society, which means that the needs of some groups go unmet. Indeed, in all of our interviews, it was an individual or group who recognized an unmet need and then worked to organize, build, and empower the community in order to fill it. Sometimes the individual or group had medical or policy expertise or access to resources, and sometimes it was a group of empowered citizens in poor communities who worked to develop their own solutions or more effective approaches for improving community health.

The survey data also showed that some CBHOs were established by empowered community residents. These groups of community residents organized themselves to build public-private partnerships and to gather both physical and less tangible social capital forms of resources to support programs to improve community health outcomes. Where this occurred, a careful examination of both in-person interview data and the mission statements of those CBHOs illustrates their focus on meeting the health, mental health, and social support needs of groups such as the uninsured, the poor, immigrants, and the various racial and ethnic communities that have customarily been disempowered in U.S. society.

The symbolic interaction approach strongly urges greater understanding among people in their interactions. This approach is in keeping with the many opportunities for interaction created by the activities of CBHOs as they organize, build, and empower their community for health improvement. Community needs assessment, client feedback regarding quality of services, client surveys and focus groups, and even such simple measures as comment cards are all examples of interaction with the community. This concerted effort to obtain and use input from clients is evidence of the ability of CBHOs to foster interaction between clients and providers. Input from the community increases understanding between providers and consumers of service; it provides a basis on which to design provider training and to make the kinds of programmatic changes that serve to enhance service delivery.

In the symbolic interaction paradigm, this process of seeking input from their constituents places CBHOs in the position of engaging in community organizing and building by creating opportunities for providers and community members to work together. As these various kinds of stakeholders collaborate to improve health outcomes, they help build up social capital—the stock of trust and commitment and sense of responsibility and ownership of both community problems and solutions—among residents and their service providers. This collective effort, spearheaded by the local CBHO, leads to social cohesion and the development of a sense, particularly among community residents, of their ability to engage not only in "power to" but also in "power with" their partners.

From the perspective of ecological theory, community organizing and building are required at multiple levels and in the various systems within the social ecology of a community to foster change that will in turn lead to improved health. To that end, most CBHOs developed various methods of communicating with clients, policymakers, and the public at large. One effective method is community meetings and programs that serve as forums where CBHOs communicate with the public, including elected officials.

When these theoretical explanations are taken together, they suggest that CBHOs can serve as a base for organizing, building, and empowering community at multiple levels from clients to elected officials to other organizations. Ultimately, these theories point to CBHOs not only as change agents but also more as catalysts for systemic, communitywide health improvement.

Evidence of the overall effort by CBHOs to obtain input and feedback from clients and to use that information to make changes in internal operations is indeed very encouraging. However, the evidence that CBHOs play a critical role in community organizing and building, at multiple levels, suggests that there are two areas of focus that would increase the power of these organizations: services to immigrant clients and relationships with policymakers. With regard to the first area, services to immigrant clients, CBHOs would do well to include work that focuses on organizing and empowerment, which can serve to assist recent newcomers in more quickly becoming active participants in U.S. society and the democratic process. The other area has to do with the need for CBHOs to pay even more attention to their relationships with policymakers and to fine-tune their advocating skills, which are critical aspects of improving health outcomes in their communities. Advocacy and policy input have now become central to the sustainability of CBHOs. Chapter Five is devoted to a full analysis of how CBHOs will need to proceed in this area going forward.

Finally, the most pressing question for the future of CBHOs is, What are the attributes that help a CBHO maintain organizational stability and growth over time? This research provides evidence that most of the CBHOs surveyed have taken well-planned measures to remain stable and to secure their operations in various ways. They have revised mission statements when necessary, and they have sought community input and used it to train staff, guide grant writing, conduct quality management reviews and modifications in service delivery, and develop new programs. They are also seeking expansion of funding, and they are working diligently to diversify their funding streams, including instituting and collecting fees, however minimal, from patients.

Limitations of the Study

This study must be considered an introduction to the broad-based, interdisciplinary research that is needed to fully document and support the significant work being done by local CBHOs to improve health in their communities. As an introductory effort, the study was undertaken without any outside funding, and that immediately set limits on its scope.

Our primary concern was with data based on responses to surveys that were mailed to potential respondents electronically. Although the customary protocols of identification of the appropriate staff person to respond to the survey and prenotification were followed, and the target response rate was exceeded, the resulting pool of sixty-five respondents was low compared to the initial mailing of five hundred, which limited generalizability of the results to the universe of CBHOs. Finally, time did not allow for further analysis of the data, which might provide further insight into the operations of the CBHOs that participated in this study.

Preliminary Conclusions: Best Practices and Lessons Learned

Results from this study suggest that CBHOs are already working at strengthening the organizational capability of both their internal operations and their external relationships. These results are encouraging, especially for smaller CBHOs. However, none of the organizations in this study that were started in the past decade have budgets over $5 million. In the course of conducting the six in-depth interviews, this low level of funding for organizations with a ten-year track record of accomplishment was attributed by some to a clear pattern established since the 1980s of a decline in the availability of funding. Others saw their lower level of funding, despite successfully managed programs, as attributable to the economic downturn of the early 2000s, which they expected would be a relatively short-term problem.

Although the reasons for the smaller budgets of more recently established CBHOs are uncertain, it seems to indicate that as CBHOs plan for the future, one of the best practices they must employ is to rethink and tighten the connecting threads of funding and programming. Some CBHOs have already assessed this situation and taken steps to address it by increasing patient volume or charging fees. The concern, of course, is that these practices may serve as barriers to access to services for some patients. Therefore, the recommendation is to institute client fees with extreme caution, if at all.

The lesson learned here is that past efforts over the course of more than five decades to institute policies that would ensure health care for all in the United States have not been as fruitful as desired. Neither has there been a concerted effort to establish cultural and linguistically appropriate health services across all systems of health care in the nation. The result has been a history of health disparities, because without coverage or without access to culturally compatible services, some people will opt not to seek health care. Therefore, unless there is some form of universal health insurance, coupled with a concerted effort to deliver culturally sensitive services, depending on fees for service may not be an effective long-term strategy, as most of the CBHOs in the study serve populations that are overwhelmingly uninsured, poor, and immigrant.

Consequently, CBHOs now more than ever must devote a portion of their efforts to acquiring new skills and best practices that equip them to engage more strategically in advocacy and political participation as methods for empowering community, forging equal partnerships, and improving negotiating capability. There has never been a better time for these new directions because there is now greater public recognition that CBHOs and other community-based entities play a crucial role in disease prevention and control. It is hoped that thanks to this recognition, they will be considered full partners in the public health equation (Klein, Birkhead, and Murphy, 1998).

Indeed, the literature suggests that external relationships are critical to the future of CBHOs, because even competing nonprofits will have to develop functional collaborations that allow them to work on the specific health issues identified by the community (York and Zychlinski, 1996). Although it is widely acknowledged that CBHOs can effectively reach medically underserved populations, they do so by building community ties and linkages and by organizing a community around a mission, such as health, that has broad community impact (Denham, Crouse Quinn, and Gamble, 1998; Derose and others, 2000). Community organizing, however, usually involves tailoring the approach and strategies to the needs of a particular neighborhood, which often requires a multipronged approach that can include neighbors reaching out to neighbors, door-to-door outreach, the use of culturally sensitive materials for education, and ethnic media, peer support, child care, and transportation assistance (Donovan, 1997).

The difficulty is that while these are organizing activities, practices, and skills that help build and empower community, it is not easy to accurately measure of this type of work. The good news is that CBHOs are developing the technological capacity to collect, store, and retrieve data that can be used as measures of the work they do. Measuring the impact of these multiple service delivery strategies is now a necessity in order to compete for scarce funding (Light, 2000; Schlesinger, 1987) or for clients who are now being mandated to Medicaid Managed Care organizations in different parts of the country. Readily retrievable data are also critical to the management of internal operations and broader external relationships (Savitch and Kantor, 2003).

The CBHOs in this study are clearly providing a variety of services to large populations at some sites, and in that capacity they serve as the primary provider for a majority of their clients. The centrality of CBHOs to the communities they serve, as well as their current status in terms of internal operations and external relationships, has led to several suggestions for improving not only the way that CBHOs function but also their conducting their own research to evaluate the impact of their work on improving health outcomes.

Key Points

- The theoretical underpinnings of this study support the idea that CBHOs are catalytic agents in organizing, building social capital and social cohesion, and empowering communities to advocate for the kinds of changes both internally and in relationship to government and policy that can improve health outcomes.
- All CBHOs simultaneously work on organizing, building, and empowering the communities in which they operate while also delivering services. However, they must now develop more strategic ways of doing this work if they are to

effectively advocate for resources and services to improve community health.

- Some CBHOs have developed stronger relationships than others with their clients and larger community, but they all understand the need for doing this.
- Community residents, health care providers, and other stake-holders must work together to establish and operate CBHOs that provide service and simultaneously organize, build, and engage the community in strong partnerships that can advocate for improved community health.
- CBHOs must now begin to conduct their own research to evaluate the impact and effectiveness of the programs they offer.
- Interdisciplinary research on CBHOs has to increase so as not only to document the significant work being done in these organizations but also to support and justify the need for continued funding.

Study Question

You are interested in helping returning soldiers from the Iraq and Afghan wars, suffering from posttraumatic distress, who together with their families are at risk of substance abuse and its sequelae, such as homelessness and a lack of preventive health care. You decide to start an organization focused on this. Do the following:

1. Develop a mission statement.
2. Visit a local CBHO providing health, mental health, and social support services to determine the geographical community being served, the services being provided for that specific community, and sources of funding for the services and programs that CBHO is providing.
3. Identify some potential health care institutions that you would want to partner with in developing your CBHO, and explain why they are to be considered for partnerships and what they would bring to the partnership.

References
Abramson, A. J., and Salamon, L. M. *The Nonprofit Sector and the New Federal Budget*. Washington, D.C.: Urban Institute Press, 1986.

Alexander, J. "The Impact of Devolution on Nonprofits: A Multiphase Study of Social Service Organizations." *Nonprofit Management and Leadership,* 1999, *10,* 57–70.

Alexander, J., Nank, R., and Stivers, C. "Implications of Welfare Reform: Do Nonprofit Survival Strategies Threaten Civil Society?" *Nonprofit and Voluntary Sector Quarterly,* 1999, *28,* 452–475.

Bayne Smith, M. A. "Ethnic Organizations and the Politics of Multiculturalism: The Case of Caribbean Americans." *Research in Social Policy,* 1996, *4,* 145–171.

Below, P. J., Morrisey, G. L, and Acomb, B. L. *The Executive Guide to Strategic Planning.* San Francisco: Jossey-Bass, 1987.

Brager, G., Specht, H., and Torczyner, J. L. *Community Organizing.* (2nd ed.) New York: Columbia University Press, 1987.

Bureau of Primary Health Care. *Models That Work: A Compendium of Innovative Primary Health Care Programs for Underserved and Vulnerable Populations.* Bethesda, Md.: Bureau of Primary Health Care, 1996.

Denham, A., Crouse Quinn, S., and Gamble, D. "Community Organizing for Health Promotion in the Rural South: An Exploration of Community Competence (Community Interventions)." *Family and Community Health,* 1998, *21,* 1–21.

Derose, K. P., and others. "Dealing with Diversity: Recruiting Churches and Women for a Randomized Trial of Mammography Promotion." *Health Education and Behavior,* 2000, *27,* 632–648.

Donovan, J. "A Question of Community: At Not-for-Profit Hospitals, Health Is a Local Affair." *Fund Raising Management,* 1997, *28*(8), 32–36.

Halpern, R. *Rebuilding the Inner City: A History of Neighborhood Initiatives to Address Poverty in the United States.* New York: Columbia University Press, 1995.

Irigoyen, M., and Findley, S. E. "Methodological Difficulties in Assessing Contributions by Community-Based Organizations to Improving Child Health." Editorial. *Archives of Pediatric and Adolescent Medicine,* 1998, *152,* 318–320.

Klein, S. J., Birkhead, G. S., and Murphy, D. P. "Role of Community-Based Organization in Control of Sexually Transmitted Diseases." Letter to the editor. *Journal of the American Medical Association,* 1998, *280,* 419.

Light, P. C. *Making Nonprofits Work: A Report on the Tides of Nonprofit Management Reform.* Washington, D.C.: Brookings Institution Press, 2000.

Lynn, P., Beerten, R., Laiho, J., and Martin, J. *Recommended Standard Final Outcome Categories and Standard Definitions of Response Rate for Social Surveys.* Colchester, England: Institute for Social and Economic Research, 2001.

McKenzie, J. F., Pinger, R. R., and Kotecki, J. E. *An Introduction to Community Health.* Boston: Jones & Bartlett, 2002.

Minkler, M. "Introduction and Overviews." In M. Minkler (ed.), *Community Organizing and Community Building for Health*. New Brunswick, N.J.: Rutgers University Press, 2002.

Nadel, M. V. *Community Health Centers: Challenges in Transitioning to Prepaid Managed Care*. Publication HEHS-95-143. Gaithersburg, Md.: General Accounting Office, 1995.

Reagan, P. A., and Brookins-Fisher, J. *Community Health in the 21st Century*. Upper Saddle River, N.J.: Prentice Hall, 2002.

Rohde, J., and Wyon, J. *Community-Based Health Care: Lessons from Bangladesh to Boston*. Boston: Management Sciences for Health, 2002.

Salamon, L. M. "The Crisis of the Nonprofit Sector and the Challenge of Renewal." *National Civic Review*, 1996, *85*(4), 3–16.

Savitch, H. V., and Kantor, P. "Urban Strategies for a Global Era: A Cross-National Comparison." *American Behavioral Scientist*, 2003, *46*, 1002–1033.

Schauffler, H. H., and Wolin, J. "Community Health Clinics Under Managed Care Competition: Navigating Uncharted Waters." *Journal of Health Politics, Policy and Law*, 1996, *21*, 461–488.

Schlesinger, M. "Paying the Price: Medical Care, Minorities, and the Newly Competitive Health Care System." *Milbank Quarterly*, 1987, *65*, 271–295.

Schlesinger, M., Gray, B., and Bradley, E. "Charity and Community: The Role of Nonprofit Ownership in a Managed Health Care System." *Journal of Health Politics, Policy and Law*, 1996, *21*, 697–751.

Sheehan, K. B., and McMillan, S. J. "Response Variation in E-Mail Surveys: An Exploration." *Journal of Advertising Research*, 1999, *39*(4), 45–54.

Wells, B. L., and Conviser, R. "Evaluating the Elimination of Disparities: Issues and Approaches to Health Status and Outcomes Assessment." *Journal of Health Education*, 1998, *29*(5), S6–S22.

Witmer, A., and others. "Community Health Workers: Integral Members of the Health Care Workforce." *American Journal of Public Health*, 1995, *85*, 1055–1058.

Wolf, T. *Managing a Nonprofit Organization in the Twenty-First Century*. New York: Simon & Schuster, 1999.

Wurzbach, M. E. *Community Health Education and Promotion: A Guide to Program Design and Evaluation*. Gaithersburg, Md.: Aspen, 2002.

York, A., and Zychlinski, E. "Competing Nonprofit Organizations Also Collaborate." *Nonprofit Management and Leadership*, 1996, *7*, 15–27.

Chapter Four

Case Study: The Health Keepers Model of Service Delivery

Yvonne J. Graham

This chapter presents a case study of a New York City community-based health organization (CBHO), the Caribbean Women's Health Association, Inc., and its method of service delivery, the Health Keepers Model. This case study draws on more than twenty years of experience to explain a model that is capable of significant community penetration, involvement, and development. It also describes why this model is effective when employed by small, local entities. The chapter concludes by offering some possible new approaches CBHOs could consider to strengthen their capacity to adjust to the broader forces of politics, economics, cultural trends, immigration, and community needs.

Learning Objectives

- An understanding of the health beliefs and practices of a particular population is a key element in assessing contributing factors for disparities and in planning interventions to increase the ability of the population to gain access to and use the health care system.

- When health is defined from a community perspective, approaches to care go beyond the limits of the traditional biomedical model of disease, the patient, etiology, and treatment, to include the underlying causes of diseases, perceptions of health and illness, and delivery and use of health care within a community's cultural, social, economic, and geopolitical milieu.
- Because poor health is closely associated with low socioeconomic status, any attempt to address the health care needs of a population must provide families with economic opportunities, social networks, and services that help them find and remain in decent and affordable housing, keep their children in school and help them succeed, obtain jobs that pay a living wage, provide a career path, secure health and social services, build assets and create wealth, and contribute to the revitalization of their neighborhoods.
- Services to ethnic and immigrant populations are more effective when they are neighborhood-based; when community members are included in the assessment of needs and the design, development, implementation, and evaluation of programs; and when services are integrated and comprehensive in scope.
- Pitfalls in government funding, such as lack of support for organizational infrastructure and contracting delays, limit the ability of CBHOs to provide needed services.
- To survive the vicissitudes associated with government contracts, CBHOs must consider alternative mechanisms to ensure sustainability.

Responding to Immigrants' Needs: A Contextual Overview

In 1982, the Caribbean Women's Health Association, Inc. (CWHA), a community-based organization, was established as a result of the failure of mainstream service delivery systems and institutions to provide appropriate services for the large Caribbean immigrant population in New York City. Simultaneously, a conference on health and Caribbean immigrants in New York City was convened in connection with a doctoral dissertation, "The Development of a Framework for Health Care Advocacy on Behalf of Caribbean Immigrants" (Mason,

1985). The conference brought together scholars, health policy-makers, and community leaders to formulate strategies to address the health care, immigration, and social service needs of this burgeoning population. It concluded with a consensus mandate to create and institutionalize a formal structure to advocate on behalf of Caribbean immigrants and respond to their needs through population-specific interventions. CWHA adopted this mandate as it formalized its corporate identity.

During that same time, there was increased recognition of the alarming differences in health status between minority and non-minority populations in the United States. One indication was the report released by the Task Force on Black and Minority Health, an initiative of the secretary of Health and Human Services (Heckler, 1985). The task force studied black, Hispanic, Native American, and Asian and Pacific Islander communities. The report highlighted six specific health areas that accounted for more than 80 percent of the higher annual proportion of minority deaths: cardiovascular and cerebrovascular diseases; cancer; chemical dependency; diabetes; homicide, suicide, and unintentional injuries; and infant mortality and low birth weight.

The most striking differentials noted in the report were the gap of more than five years in life expectancy between blacks and whites and the infant mortality rate, which for blacks was twice that of whites (Malone and Johnson, 1986). The task force further identified a variety of factors that limit accessibility to health services, including language differences, low socioeconomic status, psychological barriers, and lack of trained personnel serving minority communities. These issues were not new to ethnic community-based health organizations (CBHOs) like CWHA that served primarily immigrants. But the report supported their position that there was a critical need to address health disparities by identifying contributing factors and instituting targeted interventions that would improve access to health care.

Concurrently, research conducted by the New York City Department of Health indicated that during the years 1980–1984, black women in New York City had a maternal mortality rate five times that of white women and more than twice that of other racial groups (Chavkin, 1985). Wendy Chavkin pointed out that among this black population, a surprisingly high maternal mortality rate was exhibited by the Caribbean subpopulation. Further, she reported that infant mortality rates among the city's immigrant Caribbean population were excessive when compared both to other immigrant groups and to American blacks, whites, and Hispanics.

Also during that same period, research studies conducted at two local area hospitals in Brooklyn, New York, found that among low-income Caribbean immigrants, particularly Haitians, cancer of the cervix was more likely to be detected in the advanced stages than it was among U.S.-born black women in Brooklyn (Fruchter, Boyce, and Hunt, 1980). According to Rachel Fruchter, community surveys and screening programs conducted in association with the studies validated that immigrant women were less likely than U.S.-born black women to have had a Pap test for cancer of the cervix, do breast self-examination, and have regular medical care. Among the reasons cited by the study were lack of timely and preventive health care to arrest or treat the disease at an early stage and barriers in accessing care.

These research reports strengthened CWHA's advocacy for population-specific approaches to health service delivery. These approaches revolved around the establishment and operation of neighborhood-based structures to help new immigrants adjust to their new host environment and help constituents access needed health, immigration, and social support services.

In response to increased immigration and the AIDS epidemic, a number of similar organizations emerged around that time. Some were set up primarily to respond to the AIDS epidemic (such as the Center for an Urban Future) and others to address immigrants' acculturation and economic self-sufficiency issues (Leicher, 2001). Some of these organizations were run exclusively by volunteers and were largely connected to religious institutions. Others, like CWHA, were sufficiently developed to attract government and foundation grants. However, all were instrumental in providing a range of services to high-risk families through such means as outreach, education and counseling, home visiting, advocacy, and translation.

The role that ethnic associations play in their communities gave them a clear identity. Their distinguishing characteristics were their understanding of the intricate cultural system of new immigrant populations, the sociopolitical dynamics of the communities they serve, and their strategic position as a bridge between ethnic communities and mainstream medical systems. In addition to these functions, ethnic associations had a reputation as a trusted resource for residents, providing education and advice on the political, educational, law enforcement, and health care systems. It is these essential functions that formed the framework for the development of the Health Keepers Model.

The Health Keepers Model is based on several assumptions. The first assumption is that health must be defined from a community perspective, which requires that care go beyond the limits of the traditional biomedical model of disease to equally focus on the underlying cause of diseases, perception of health and illness, and delivery and utilization of health care within a community's cultural, social, economic, and geopolitical milieu.

Therefore, examining the relationship among health, ethnicity, and cultural issues as they relate to delivery and acceptance of health care in immigrant communities is a critical dimension in planning services for those populations (Kleinman, Eisenberg, and Good, 1978). In addition, a broad understanding of the historical, demographic, socioeconomic, and political context of a community is important in determining the types of policies, programs, and institutions that are best suited to address the health care needs of its residents. This is particularly relevant in large urban and poor communities where cultural diversity has become the defining characteristic in planning for health care services.

The second assumption is that poor health is closely associated with low socioeconomic status and low levels of educational attainment (Mason, 1985). Any attempt to improve health status must therefore involve soliciting communitywide input in problem identification and formulation and implementation of strategies that will help community members move from poverty to self-sufficiency. As discussed in Chapter Two, Paulo Freire in his book *Pedagogy of the Oppressed* (1990) suggests that when individuals are able to identify the root cause of problems, they tend to take greater responsibility in making changes that will be beneficial to their health. Some of the strategies that can lead to empowerment and self-sufficiency include the following:

- Community involvement in identifying issues and planning for change
- Providing economic opportunities to increase self-reliance

- Connecting individuals and families to social networks and services that help them find and remain in decent and affordable housing, keep their children in school, and help them succeed in their studies
- Providing jobs that pay a living wage
- Helping families identify and pursue a career path
- Teaching individuals how to build assets, create wealth, and contribute to the revitalization of their neighborhoods

Many of these initiatives do not typically fall within the domain of mainstream health care institutions, but as mentioned earlier, they are the defining characteristics of CBHOs. In fact, an article published by the New York Regional Association of Grantmakers titled "Responding to Immigrant Needs" stated that many new immigrants reported that they are not always well served by large social services agencies and that it takes longer for the large agencies to make the connection (Siska, 2002). For these reasons and others, fund collaborators expressed a commitment to helping community-based organizations with capacity building to develop their administrative and leadership capability so that they can help increase access to government benefits and services (Siska, 2002).

The third assumption is that services to underserved and immigrant populations are more effective when they are neighborhood-based; when community members are included in assessment of needs, design, development, implementation, and evaluation of programs; and when services are comprehensive in scope (Center for New York City Affairs, 2003).

These assumptions provide the contextual background on which CWHA was founded and the domain within which it functions.

The Caribbean Community

Cultural diversity has played a major role in New York City's reputation as the international capital of the world. By 1985, the population of the United States had become more ethnically plural than ever before, and this was most evident in its large urban centers such as New York City (Bogen, 1985). For example, according to the 2000 census, Caribbean immigrants represent a significant proportion—approximately one-third—of New York City's foreign-born residents (New York City Department of City Planning, 2002). Since their arrival in the early 1900s, they have filled labor needs, contributed to the city's economic vibrancy, and enriched the cultural fabric of the city. Despite these contributions, Caribbean people, like many other immigrants, are often the lowest-paid workers, facing language barriers and lacking access to basic services. One of the outcomes of these conditions is poor health, most notable in data released by the New York City Department of Health and Mental Hygiene. These data show higher infant mortality rates and higher mortality and morbidity from HIV/AIDS and a greater incidence of childhood asthma, certain forms of cancer, and chronic health conditions in neighborhoods where Caribbean people are concentrated.

Federal, state, and local governments have supported initiatives that seek to improve access to care and health insurance coverage and to facilitate language competency in low-income and largely immigrant populations. However, as the city's share of foreign-born residents continues to spiral upward, and as the city encounters the greatest financial crisis in decades, public health systems and local communities face the challenge of finding more effective ways of addressing health disparities among racial and ethnic minorities. In so doing, much emphasis has been placed on local community action on the premise that local communities can have the greatest impact on health by serving as a bridge between residents and mainstream service systems. In this role, they develop and implement strategies for creation and dissemination of health information and health education messages and serve as facilitators in using mainstream services.

The New York State Public Health Council's report "Communities Working Together for a Healthier New York" (1996) indicated that the key to improving the health of New Yorkers is the community aspect of community health. Understanding the community and involving community residents are vital to appropriate assessment, program planning, and targeting of resources and provides a strong advocacy base for community health. Community involvement empowers individuals and motivates them to engage in communitywide action to address specific problems. This, in turn, promotes community ownership of health conditions, improves the general welfare of its residents, and builds social capital. To effectively engage a community and leverage its resources, an inventory must be made of its residents, organizations, stakeholders, and human and health service delivery systems.

Community mapping is one of the most important ways of gathering information for health policymakers, funders, and health providers to use in allocating resources and targeting health outreach and educational interventions. Community mapping entails an assessment of the physical makeup of the community; the demographic, social, and economic characteristics of its residents; their religious and cultural beliefs, family structure, and the role of the family in health service use; their attitude toward the service delivery system; and any other factors associated with access to care. It also includes an examination of the political system, leaders, and resource agencies in the community.

For purposes of this discussion, the Caribbean immigrant population in the borough of Brooklyn, New York, will be used as a case study. This group has all the ingredients for a good case study. First of all, Brooklyn is home to the largest concentration of Caribbean immigrants in the United States. This population has emigrated in large numbers for almost four decades and has established strong community roots. Second, we now have sufficient epidemiological data on this population from which to make inferences or draw conclusions. It is also a culturally diverse population, which lends itself to a wide-ranging discussion of health beliefs and practices, religion, language differences, and socioeconomic status and of how these factors influence attitudes and behaviors and impede access to care. Further, it is the primary target group served by CWHA and in which the Health Keepers Model was developed.

History

The Caribbean region includes all the island nations of the Caribbean Sea and the nations of Central America from Belize to Panama—thirty-five nations in all. It is important to underscore that the Caribbean population is far from a homogenous group. This diversity is a result of the colonization of the various territories by France, England, Spain, and Holland during the slave trade. They have many different cultures, ethnic groups, languages, educational systems, religious beliefs, and practices. But the majority share an African ancestry.

The historical significance of the Caribbean region is great. It was the first important European overseas experiment with capitalism, the starting place for tropical overseas agriculture better known as the plantation system, and a primary site of large-scale enslavement of African peoples in the New World (Mintz, 1974). After the abolition of slavery, its position became one of strategic military importance to the United States, and the region is popularly known as the "third border" of the United States.

The social structure of Caribbean people is deeply rooted in the history of slavery, plantation life, and colonialism. During the slave trade, individuals were forcibly taken from their communities in Africa, their family structures were destroyed, their religions were not respected in their new land, and they suffered immeasurably at the hands of their masters. Many generations later, most of these territories achieved independence from their colonial masters. The governments of the newly independent territories fell along a spectrum from free and democratic states to ones that favored a ruling class with little opportunity for the masses to become upwardly mobile. Others, such as Haiti, endured an oligarchy for many decades (Antoine, 1985).

The presence of Caribbean people in the United States dates back to the 1920s, when a mostly professional working-class group of immigrants settled among native-born blacks and quickly became assimilated into the larger black population (Thomas, 1977). A second wave arrived as a result of the 1965 immigration law, which allowed increased immigration from that region. Unlike the previous wave, the great majority of these new immigrants were unskilled laborers seeking greater economic opportunities and upward mobility. Over the years, they have established strong economic and cultural roots in the communities where they settled, changing the ethnic character of those neighborhoods.

Demographics

Over the past two decades, the nation as a whole has undergone a demographic shift. The 2000 census indicates that minority residents (African Americans, Hispanics, Asians, Native Americans, and other racial and ethnic minorities) now account for nearly half the population of the nation's largest cities. New York City has historically been recognized as the Mecca for immigrants from around the world and is considered the most culturally diverse place on earth. This tradition continues as evidenced by census data showing that New York City's share of foreign-born residents increased from 28.4 percent in 1990 to 35.9 percent in 2000. In contrast, the native-born population declined from 71.6 percent in 1990 to 64.1 percent in 2000.

There are approximately 1.9 million persons of Caribbean ancestry in the United States, according to the 2000 census; 725,000 of them reside in New York State, 589,000 in New York City, and 297,000 in Brooklyn (U.S. Census Bureau, 2003). This represents nearly 12 percent of Brooklyn's 2.5 million people and constitutes the largest concentration of Caribbean immigrants in the country. This figure does not take into account persons who are undocumented, which estimates place at anywhere from 50,000 to 250,000.

Geographical Boundaries

In New York City, Caribbean people are concentrated in specific neighborhoods. The largest concentration is in central Brooklyn, where they have established strong cultural, social, and economic roots. This is evident in their level of home ownership, businesses, transportation system, churches, financial institutions, civic and cultural associations, community-based health and social service organizations, and immigration centers. In addition, they have their own ethnic print and electronic media sources that provide information and services that are culturally relevant and language-appropriate.

Socioeconomics

The Caribbean population in New York City is a vibrant, productive, and ambitious group of people. They contribute significantly to the stability, economic growth, and cultural fabric of the city. The annual West Indian Carnival and Labor Day Parade in Brooklyn attracts more than 3.5 million people and adds an estimated $2 million to the city's coffers. Many Caribbean families are middle-class, owners of businesses, professionals, and upwardly mobile. But a large proportion is unskilled, and many, particularly those from French- and Spanish-speaking territories such as Haiti and the Dominican Republic, are unable to speak English well. As a result, they have difficulty finding good-paying jobs.

Persons with little or no technical skills and those for whom language is a barrier tend to find employment in small ethnic community businesses where English-language proficiency and technical knowledge are not required. One of the downsides of this is that small employers are unable to pay competitive salaries or to offer employment-based health insurance. As a result, these individuals have difficulty accessing health care services and are subject to the social ills and adverse health outcomes that beset the poor.

Health Indicators

Overall, the population in the United States experienced a decline in death rates from all causes over the past three decades. The decline in infant mortality during this period is unparalleled by other mortality reductions in the past century ("Achievements in Public Health," 1999). This is largely due to progress in understanding the causes and risks for developing diseases; in the capacity of medicine to diagnose, treat, and cure diseases; in the long-term management of chronic diseases; and in behavioral science research and methodology. Despite these advances, certain minority groups, including immigrants from the Caribbean region, continue to show a distressing disparity in key health indicators. Chief among these are measures of maternal and child health, which are key indicators in assessing the health status of a community. For example, the New York City Department of Health in a 2002 report indicated that despite a citywide average in infant mortality rate (IMR) of 6.9 per thousand live births, there were population subgroups in the city for whom infant mortality rates were far higher than the citywide average. It was determined that the ethnic groups with the highest IMRs in New York City were predominantly from a dozen countries in the circum-Caribbean region (Freiden, 2002).

In response to these data and to gain a better understanding of the problem, a number of focus groups were conducted to elicit information and perceptions from women in the identified groups regarding what they saw as some of the contributing factors to the high IMRs for their group. The two major themes that repeatedly surfaced throughout the discussions revolved around systemic and institutional issues of access to health care and culturally influenced beliefs and health behaviors. A striking aspect of all the explanations offered was the underlying connecting thread of poverty and the need not only for comprehensive programs and services that respond to the immediate medical need but also for strategies to help families move from poverty to self-sufficiency.

Religion

Spirituality is one of the most profound aspects of black culture and has a significant influence on behavior. Caribbean people embrace a wide range of religious faiths, with Catholic, Protestant, and Pentecostal denominations in the majority. There are many who also simultaneously practice ancestral religions as part of traditional practices brought to these lands from Africa during slavery. In Haiti, for example, people practice Catholicism and do not see a conflict with vodou because they see vodou not only as an ancestral religion but also as a way of life. Vodou practices are embedded in the family, cultural expressions, literature, the performing arts, housebuilding, planting, harvesting, and health and illness (Frank, 2001).

Similarly, Santeria practiced in Spanish-speaking territories, contrary to popular belief, is a benevolent religious practice and should not be equated with sorcery or "black magic." To bear out this point in the health care context, a traditional Haitian herbalist or a physician can treat a person who suffers from asthma, fever, or the common cold because these types of illnesses are categorized as "God's malady" and are caused by natural forces. On the contrary, illnesses thought to be from supernatural causes, such as mental illness, may result from neglect of one's protective guide assigned at birth. To bring back harmony, the voodoo priest or priestess is the healer of choice (Frank, 2001). HIV/AIDS prevention and treatment has also presented formidable challenges in instances where the cause of the illness is attributed to "Satan's malady," arising from the revenge of an enemy who wants to destroy the individual. In this case, after falling ill, the individual often consults with the voodoo priest or priestess for treatment rather than seek the services of a medical doctor.

Other instances where religion affects health care involve pregnancy planning, abortion, sexual relationships before marriage, and domestic violence. The issue of domestic violence deserves special mention in that precincts serving large numbers of people from the Caribbean report an excessive number of police interventions for domestic altercations (Office of the District Attorney, 2002). In this sense, religions that promote women's obedience to their husbands can be seen as a contributing factor.

Health Beliefs and Practices

The health beliefs and practices of Caribbean people are a mixture of traditional folk health and mainstream medical systems. Although one cannot generalize about the use of traditional folk healers and Western medical practices or a combination thereof, providers should become familiar with the different sectors of their health care system (popular, folk, and biomedical) and the interface between these systems. The use of one or all of these systems and the choice of health providers can be different for each person, depending on his or her beliefs or social class. Most middle-class Caribbean immigrants use the mainstream Western medical systems because services are more financially accessible, but they are not the majority of immigrants. The majority of Caribbean people who migrated after 1965 came from working-class and lower-class backgrounds. Given the difficulties associated with obtaining good-paying jobs that offer health insurance, they often rely on cheaper and more readily available folk medicine. Upon migrating, some immigrants assimilate and adopt the culture of their new environment. Others retain their beliefs and attitudes when they migrate to the United States, and this influences their concepts of health and illness and hence their use of health care services.

Literature on illness behavior suggests that variation in the practice of folk health within groups based on class, religious practices, and beliefs is much greater than it is between groups and that social class in particular plays an important role (McLaughlin, 1985). How one defines and expresses illness and the help that one seeks are to a large extent shaped by sociocultural factors. That substantial segments of Caribbean populations continue to rely on these alternative therapies is evident by the number of *botanicas* dispersed throughout the community, offering herbal and alternative treatments.

Folk healers do good business in the United States because their model of care closely resembles that of the home country of the immigrant, not only in the treatment modality but also in the nature of the relationship between provider and patient or family. Western medical services tend to be very formal, whereas touching and family involvement characterize folk healing. In addition, folk healers are usually members of the community, and their services are viewed as cheaper, more relevant to their clients, and less bureaucratic. Further, their approach to health care is both reactive and proactive, rather than primarily reactive, as is the case with Western medicine. Folk healers are also very responsive in providing services designed to "protect" their patients from any anticipated foul play or potential harm.

Despite the use of folk healers when there are suspicions of potential physical illness, primary and preventive health care is not used as much as it should be by many Caribbean people. Further, preventive health care in particular is sometimes not well understood in the Caribbean community. Among those who rely on traditional folk medicine, beliefs about the treatment of diseases are grounded in theories regarding the etiology of the illness. For example, if the source of the disease or illness is thought to arise from supernatural sources, traditional healers would be the primary persons sought for this ailment. On the other hand, if the etiology is perceived as stemming from physical causes, a physician would be sought for treatment (Frank, 1985).

It is important to note that not all Caribbean cultures are alike and not all people in or from a given country will exhibit the same health behaviors. As stated earlier, health behavior is mediated not only by culture but also largely by social class. Nevertheless, many ailments, such as the common cold, flu, high blood pressure, and asthma, are often treated with herbs and teas, in some cases combined with a medical regimen. Because of the potential danger for adverse reactions from combining medications, it is important that providers determine whether patients are taking home remedies. Patients are often reluctant to reveal this kind of information to persons outside of their culture or do not consider home remedies as medication.

While it is important not to lose sight of the influence of class, there is a tendency for health issues to be handled within the family, with family members having distinct roles. In these situations, certain family members may serve as decision makers or support or reinforce health behaviors. Pregnancy, for example, is often thought of as a state of being, not a medical condition, and common discomforts of pregnancy are handled by family members. Health practices during pregnancy may entail using certain tcas made from the bark and leaves of trees to cleanse the inside of the body. Fish broth is taken to strengthen the body, and sex during pregnancy is considered vital to strengthening the baby. Starch and okra are eaten to facilitate the birth process. Medical aid is sought for severe complications and for childbirth (Browne, Graham, and Hylton, 1986).

As families become more acculturated in subsequent generations, they are less likely to rely on the extended family and more likely to adapt to mainstream service delivery systems. However, there is an acknowledged shared desire to maintain ties to the cultural traditions of the home society. This is manifested in a number of ways. For example, household organization, landmark identification, values, music, and cultural beliefs and practices are often transplanted and maintained in the new environment. Thus like many other immigrant neighborhoods, Caribbean communities have the distinct characteristics of an ethnic enclave. This system is supported by ethnic organizations that serve to maintain cultural practices and create opportunities for families to return home permanently in the future. There is also reluctance among many immigrants to surrender their citizenship status in their birth country to become American citizens because doing so is viewed as severing ties with the home society. This reluctance has drawbacks when it comes to accessing health and social services that require citizenship status.

Family Systems and Roles

Unlike other ethnic groups, women from the Caribbean not only migrate in larger numbers than men but also tend to come first because it is easier for them to find employment (Bogen, 1985). They tend to migrate in their prime childbearing years, between the ages of fifteen and forty-four. When their male partners join them, the women have to guide them through a system that is alien to them until they are able to find work. During this period, the women are also the wage earners. This represents a complete reversal of roles. In the home country, the male is seen as the head of household and the breadwinner. The inverted situation is often very distressing to the male, especially if it takes a long time for him to find work. He may become depressed or resort to alcohol, and family conflicts may occur.

Children of immigrants also face peculiar migration-related problems. First of all, many parents leave their children behind with grandparents and other family members so that they can settle, find a home, and then reunite the family. By the time the family is reunited, the children may be adolescents or approaching adolescence. Because of the separation, they tend to have little or no emotional bond with the parents, which leads to communication difficulties, conflicts, and alienation and sometimes requires intervention. Second, many children find themselves caught between two cultures. The child-rearing techniques practiced at home may conflict with what is taught at school and practiced in the United States. For example, many Caribbean families believe in corporal punishment and in not talking about sexuality, sexually transmitted diseases, or pregnancy. This conflicts with the new culture in which the children find themselves, and the resulting problems can range from conduct disorders and juvenile delinquency to adolescent pregnancy and involvement with the child welfare system.

Seniors are also adversely affected by migration. In their home country, the elders are in charge. Young couples look to them for advice about matters such as marital relationships, childbearing, and health-related matters. In the United States, this role changes as the elders must now depend on younger family members to help them navigate the various systems. As they age, they face the possibility of living in a nursing home, a concept that is not looked on favorably in the Caribbean.

Language

The Caribbean population is multilingual and multifaceted within a given language. The major languages spoken are English, Spanish, French, and Dutch. There are also a number of dialects that are a combination of the major formal language and various African tongues. The dialects are mostly oral and are in some instances the main means of communication for individuals who are not formally educated. For individuals whose primary language is not English, their inability to speak English or to speak it well is a major barrier in accessing services in the United States. Many individuals who are not proficient in the use of the English language resort to accepting low-paying jobs in which they do not have to rely on language skills. Language barriers also restrict their ability to advance personally and to participate in their children's education.

Further, language barriers prevent parents from pursuing further educational goals, making economic progress, securing good-paying jobs, and participating fully in their children's education. According to a report on immigrant organizations conducted for United Way of New York City, many seniors often never learn to speak English, and their movement becomes limited due to their language difficulties (Leicher, 2001).

In the health care setting, it is not uncommon to see children being used as interpreters for their parents. In cultures where sensitive topics are not discussed between parents and children, it means that parents will be selective about the personal information they give to the child to convey to the doctor. This can result in misdiagnosis or inadequate treatment. Leicher (2001) also indicated that almost every provider interviewed in connection with the study recounted stories of children pulled out of school in order to help translate for parents at a clinic visit, job interview, or court appointment.

This phenomenon of the use of children in helping parents negotiate systems and, in the case of health, sensitive medical situations is worthy of further study. Of particular research interest is the question of how this practice of involving children in adult tasks, which currently occurs among newcomers, compares to the experiences of earlier immigrant groups.

Legal and Immigration Issues

In addition to sharing the same basic needs as the rest of the population, immigrants face unique barriers because of their immigration status. This is particularly evident in the areas of employment, education, and use of and entitlement to health care services. With regards to employment, many immigrants are not aware of their rights as workers and face employment discrimination. Some are offered low-paying jobs and work long hours, often in hazardous conditions and without health insurance. The undocumented, who have little or no recourse, are often victims of unscrupulous employers.

When it comes to health care, new permanent residents are prohibited from using Medicaid in the first two years of gaining that status. Therefore, they must find alternative means of paying for their health care. In addition, many naturalized citizens or permanent residents who are in the process of sponsoring relatives are reluctant to use public benefits for which they are entitled because of their fears that this may jeopardize their ability to sponsor their relatives. Further, many immigrant children who are eligible for the State Children's Health Insurance Program (SCHIP) are not enrolled because their parents may be undocumented and fear that they will be detected if they enroll their child in SCHIP. Finally, undocumented individuals shy away from services until their health condition becomes an emergency and then present themselves at a hospital emergency room.

Sources of Health Information

Sources of health information in the Caribbean immigrant community include religious leaders, community-based ethnic organizations, ethnic print and electronic media, and, to a lesser degree, mainstream systems. The decision to avail themselves of health care and their selection of a health provider depend largely on these sources. Word of mouth from community residents who have used services and found them acceptable is also a highly regarded source of health information.

Community Leaders and Resource Agencies

A distinguishing feature of immigrant communities is the visible presence of gatekeepers. Gatekeepers are individuals who operate as part of a network or individually and who understand and have influence in the political and social systems in the community. In the Caribbean immigrant community, they are often lawyers, doctors and other health professionals, religious leaders, community activists, political leaders, academicians, heads of organizations, or traditional healers. Because of their position, gatekeepers possess a certain level of credibility within the community and are relied on to protect the community's interest and preserve its culture and values. They have significant influence on the development, implementation, and acceptance of programs and services in the community and can facilitate or impede their progress.

Gatekeepers can also be very helpful in providing information about the community's values and beliefs, lifestyle, dietary habits, and other behaviors that can aid in the development of culturally appropriate interventions. The traditional healers among the most recent immigrant groups include religious types such as the santero or santera, babalao, curandero, or voodoo priest, as well as those known for their natural remedies and referred to as naturalista, yerbero, Chinese doctor, roots worker, or the like. They are all to a great extent an untapped source for information and collaboration. They possess an understanding of the cultural beliefs and practices in their communities and tend to have great influence on those who rely on their services. In this context, they should be sought out by health providers to determine how they can be included in the design, delivery, and dissemination of health education messages.

Community institutions also play a critical role in immigrant communities. Chief among them are churches and community and civic organizations. Historically, in the Caribbean community, churches have been the core institutions working to advance the well-being of residents in their constituencies. In immigrant communities, they are among the first organizations to take root, serving congregants' spiritual, social, political, and health care needs and as a clearinghouse for disseminating information (Thomas, 1977; McKnight and Kretzmann, 2002). Thomas (1977) also points out that Caribbeans tend to join associations immediately on their arrival, characterizing these associations as the lifeblood in the growth and development of their communities.

Neighborhood Issues, Local Responses

CWHA emerged as an advocacy group and service provider in the early 1980s to help immigrants adjust to their new host environment, navigate mainstream service delivery systems, and meet their cultural, legal, and linguistic needs. As health care professionals, the twelve volunteer founders of CWHA observed that many immigrants entered the health care system either for emergency treatment or when their disease was at an advanced stage with a poor prognosis. The founders recognized the need to better understand the problems immigrants face in health care use and delivery. They therefore embarked on a mission to work with policymakers, mainstream service providers, community institutions, and immigrants to develop approaches to reduce or eliminate barriers that prevent them from accessing care and improving their quality of life. The initial work of CWHA focused on health screening, counseling, and health education provided in nonthreatening environments outside the health care setting. Churches and civic organizations were natural venues, having served as traditional places of refuge for immigrants.

Early in its inception, CWHA encountered formidable challenges. One of the major challenges was the absence of reliable and comprehensive data on the health status of the Caribbean population in New York City. There was a critical need to build a strong case on which to advocate on behalf of this community. The approach was to convene a series of scholarly conferences that would yield data on Caribbean immigrants. CWHA also sought to develop a service delivery mechanism that would identify and analyze health problems and devise innovative and culturally appropriate public health interventions to improve access to care. This translated into three primary tasks:

- Building organizational leadership, organizational identity, and organizational infrastructure
- Identifying public health issues that would attract public and private support
- Identifying ways to build community consensus and facilitate community participation

It was determined that in order to assess the health care needs of the Caribbean American community and to design targeted interventions, they would first work on building relationships with New York City's health agencies, elected officials, policymakers, researchers, academicians, and service providers. This was the approach developed to collect and analyze available data, and it was accomplished via three distinct vehicles:

- A citywide health conference exploring barriers to health care delivery among immigrants
- A training seminar for service providers on delivering culturally compatible perinatal care services to immigrants

- An international and cross-cultural fact-finding field practicum for health professionals

Let's take a look at each of these initiatives in turn.

Exploring Barriers to Health Care Delivery: An Immigrant Health Conference

The health conference, titled "Delivering Health Care Services to Immigrant Communities: The Caribbean-American Experience," was held in October 1985. The conference brought together a panel of experts from health, educational, governmental, and community organizations to discuss issues from an interdisciplinary perspective toward enhancing the delivery of culturally sensitive health care. Conference topics were critical health issues (cancer, maternal and infant health, adolescent pregnancy, and social and environmental health), Caribbean folk health practices, barriers to the provision of health services, and current research findings and strategies to improve health service delivery. The conference yielded the following significant information:

- Immigrant women from the Caribbean were less likely than U.S.-born black women to have regular medical care.
- Knowledge and use of health care services, as well as health outcomes, varied among Caribbean groups.
- Infant mortality rates among New York City's immigrant Caribbean population were significantly higher than those of other immigrant groups and those of American blacks, whites, and Hispanics.
- Caribbean immigrants perceive health and illness differently enough from health providers that their perceptions warrant close examination.
- Spiritual influences assume an important role in the lives of Caribbean families.
- Etiological concepts of Caribbean persons regarding illness are related to their cultural values, especially their belief systems and practices.
- Lack of understanding among health providers of the relationship between health, cultural, and ethnic issues diminished their ability to serve immigrants effectively.

Among the conference recommendations were the following:

- Collection of specific statistical data on the health of the Caribbean population by country of origin to gain a better understanding of the health needs of each subgroup
- A fair and humane immigration policy in order to integrate minorities into the mainstream of the American health system
- Inclusion of more culturally sensitive materials relating to minorities into the curriculum of U.S. medical schools, schools of public health, and medical residency programs, allowing a better appreciation of the relationship between health and ethnicity
- Training programs for health care providers on how to work with culturally diverse populations

Delivering Culturally Competent Services to Immigrants: A Training Seminar for Providers

The training seminar, titled "Delivering Culturally Compatible Perinatal Care Services to Immigrants: The Caribbean Population in New York City," was convened in December 1986. Perinatal health was selected as a priority public health issue to be dealt with for several reasons. The Task Force on Black and Minority Health of the U.S. Department of Health and Human Services had recently released its report indicating that the two most striking differentials observed in minority health were the gap of more than five years in life expectancy between blacks and whites and the infant mortality rate, which for blacks continued to be twice that of whites (Malone and Johnson, 1986). This was particularly relevant for the Caribbean immigrant population because although specific data were not available on that population, the geographical areas in which they were concentrated had disproportionately high infant mortality rates (Chavkin, 1985). Further, prenatal care legislation was introduced by the New York state assembly to provide free prenatal care for pregnant women regardless of income or immigrant status.

The conference targeted nurses, social workers, physicians, nutritionists, counselors, and health educators, with the goal of training participating health providers to effectively deliver culturally competent perinatal care services to immigrants. The major objectives were to increase knowledge about Caribbean culture and its implications for perinatal care compliance, to provide educational materials and information, and to foster a keener understanding of the patterns of health care use and its association with pregnancy management among the Caribbean population. The conference planning committee consisted of representatives of state, city, and community agencies who were responsible for developing feasible approaches to institutionalize the conference findings and recommendations.

Several weeks prior to the conference, two key informant group sessions or focus groups were convened to provide information that would be used in the conference workshops. One consisted of immigrant clients; the other consisted of providers of perinatal services. Each group met to identify and discuss specific barriers to obtaining perinatal care and perinatal service delivery problems that affect Caribbean immigrants. The providers were enthusiastic about sharing the experiences from their respective organizations, and the immigrant clients were extremely informative in relating their personal experiences in trying to obtain prenatal care services.

Analysis of the information provided by both groups clearly showed that barriers to the receipt and delivery of perinatal care to Caribbean immigrants were legal, financial, cultural, educational, communicative, and institutional. Immigrant clients explained that the uprootedness of migration is particularly traumatic for new immigrants. It is a time when they are undergoing the stress of severing ties from their families and community and must now begin to stabilize, negotiate the housing and job markets, master the English language, and become self-sufficient so as to be able to reunite their families.

They also expressed mistrust of government and the medical system, citing the use of experimental drugs and clinical trials by superpower nations, often with disastrous sequelae, and their favored dependence on ancestral, family-managed, and community-based health systems.

The most pressing need identified by the informants was to be connected with economic opportunities, housing, affordable health care, and child care assistance. They also expressed a general fear of large institutions, to which they are unaccustomed, and the large number of staff to be dealt with before actually receiving care. In addition, the Caribbean person's perception of a doctor is a person of high status who is expected to be attired in a certain way. These health clients can therefore easily be offended by Western doctors who are more relaxed in their appearance.

Immigrants who had already settled said they felt excluded from mainstream service delivery systems. Their main frustrations were a lack of recognition and respect for their cultural norms, health beliefs, and practices; lack of culturally competent service providers to plan and deliver appropriate health education messages and promote behavior change; underutilization of ethnic print and electronic media and community institutions; lack of involvement of community groups in planning interventions targeted to them; and long waiting periods at hospitals and clinics.

Service providers, particularly those who were not of Caribbean ancestry, indicated that they experienced difficulty communicating with Caribbean immigrants even when their primary language was English. This is due to the fact that many immigrants from English-speaking territories speak English with a rhythmic cadence or a distinctive lilt. Some speak dialects that may be unfamiliar to American ears. In addition, many patients were unable to provide adequate information about their medical history. The health care panelists also reported very high rates of broken appointments and noncompliance with therapeutic regimens. In some instances, immigrants would give false addresses and telephone numbers. When asked, "What would be the most important or most valuable benefit or outcome of this conference?" providers cited the following:

- Technical assistance for institutions in providing services to immigrant women
- Attendance by a diverse group of providers and in particular those who have very little knowledge about the Caribbean population
- Identification of some of the barriers as seen by providers
- Realization on the part of providers that cultural sensitivity is needed at all levels, from admission to policymaking
- Development of institution-based expertise about cross-cultural issues, cultural compatibility, and the culture of the patients being served
- Recognition of the importance of Caribbean men in the health behavior of Caribbean women

- Building coalitions with other groups to make institutional changes

It became clear that an understanding of these issues could provide helpful insights into how Caribbean immigrants view the health care system, perceive health and illness, and use health care services. It could also serve as a framework for developing targeted health care messages and services to meet the peculiar needs of immigrants from the Caribbean and foster adherence to treatment. Therefore, the preconference strategy included using information gathered from the focus group sessions along with expert knowledge on the subject matter and practical case studies to educate and train participating health providers to provide care from a cross-cultural and practical perspective.

The conference findings revealed that perinatal care was virtually unavailable and inaccessible to Caribbean women for the following reasons:

- Ignorance of or unfamiliarity with available perinatal care services and the lack of mechanisms to effectively establish linkages with existing health care delivery systems
- Fear of detection due to legal barriers arising from the undocumented immigrant status of pregnant women and their families
- Lack of planned pregnancy programs and perinatal care informational outreach and education programs directed to Caribbean women of childbearing age
- Lack of understanding of the importance of early and continuous prenatal care, resulting in inadequate prenatal care, especially in the first trimester
- Lack of background information on the part of health care providers regarding perinatal care services and health practices in the immigrants' country of origin, resulting in the delivery of culturally incompatible perinatal care services and the immigrants' postponement or rejection of prenatal care services
- Culturally conditioned tendency for self-management approaches, reliance on folk health practices for care, and having a tradition in the country of origin of relying on a midwife rather than a physician for perinatal care services
- Substance abuse and poor nutritional intake by the expectant mother resulting in adverse effects on the developing fetus

- Economic barriers resulting from unemployment, lack of health insurance, or underinsurance

International Fact-Finding Field Practicum and Seminar

In 1988, CWHA organized the first in a series of field study tours to the Caribbean for health professionals. Participants included service providers, physicians, nurses, social workers, academicians, and health policymakers. Prior to departure, tour participants received advance information about health care in the countries to be visited and a "culture-gram" describing the country's history, government, population, lifestyle, customs, and courtesies.

The study tour included visits to hospitals, clinics, and other health care facilities. Participants also had the opportunity to take part in conferences, lectures, and panel discussions with host-country officials. A major component of the tour was a seminar specifically designed to provide a comparative interdisciplinary, transcultural, and sociomedical perspective to better understand the context of international health issues, migration, and adjustment and their implication for health service delivery. Key issues explored were how health and social services were used in the immigrants' country of origin, how they were perceived, and some elements of service delivery that might work well in immigrant communities in the United States.

The experience and information gained from the conference, the training seminar, and the international fact-finding tour provided CWHA with a vantage point from which to seek funding to assist immigrant women in accessing prenatal care. CWHA received a grant from New York State Department of Health to provide outreach to immigrant Caribbean women who were pregnant and refer them for prenatal care. At the same time, the organization confronted the challenge of building an infrastructure within which to administer the program and to conduct community-organizing efforts to ensure the success of the program. Early in this process, CWHA recognized the need to establish a model of service delivery that could be replicated in other immigrant communities. The model later became known as the Health Keepers Model.

The Health Keepers Model:
Old Concept, New Paradigms

The Health Keepers Model is a new approach to an old concept that is based on providing organized illness prevention and health promotion interventions outside of mainstream institutions. These types of community-based health services have existed in various forms for millennia. They can be found in the sick benefit societies and associations in some of the relatively sophisticated societies of early Rome and Greece. They were also the focus of the provident organizations throughout many of the northern European societies of the eighteenth and nineteenth centuries.

As early as 1880, New York City established the Division of Child Hygiene, which demonstrated that public health nurses could reduce infant mortality through home visits and health teaching. In 1883, Lillian Wald organized the Henry Street Nurses Settlement to address the health-related needs, especially of children, in the tenements of New York City.

During the early 1940s, political and economic interests resulted in a tremendous growth of the health care industry. Part of this growth was a proliferation of hospitals and a shift in the delivery of health care. Health care delivery, in large part, moved from the community-based and public health approach that centered around social and environmental factors to a biomedical approach focusing on research and technologically advanced methods of diagnosis and treatment.

By the late 1970s, it became clear that despite technological advances in medicine and increased capacity to diagnose and treat diseases, a significant proportion of the population had not benefited. This was most evident by increased documentation during the late 1970s and early 1980s of health disparities among racial and ethnic minorities (Heckler, 1985).

Among the reasons for these disparities, as cited in U.S. Department of Health and Human Services' report on black and minority health (Heckler, 1985) are the health of the mother before and during pregnancy, parental socioeconomic status, lifestyle characteristics, and immigrant issues that limit access to care. The report also made several recommendations for prevention and promotion:

- Expanding education and information services by focusing on health care delivery from a neighborhood, resident-driven, and culturally competent framework
- Addressing the needs of the whole person through an improved and comprehensive system of service delivery that integrates a range of health and social service providers and faith-based, civic, academic, and other community institutions
- Introducing legislative and regulatory measures to provide appropriate screening, patient care, and follow-up for potentially high-risk women
- Providing adequate public financing for education, outreach, and support services for women and their infants

These recommendations pointed to the need for new paradigms in delivering health care to increasingly diverse and underserved populations. It also fostered new interest in informal support systems and ethnic associations that offered alternative means of providing health services within a broader social, economic, environmental, and cultural framework. The recommendations were even more poignant because around that time period, HIV/AIDS had emerged as a new disease with behavioral and lifestyle implications. In response, a number of informal groups were set up to address the issue.

CWHA's early work as a volunteer, resident-led, grassroots community-based organization providing services to a culturally diverse population allowed it to build on this experience and develop a service delivery mechanism that could be shared with other organizations. Further, CWHA had obtained nonprofit and tax-exempt status, established an advisory board, and secured office space from which to operate. This would all eventually evolve into the Health Keepers Model.

The Health Keepers Model rests on three ideological principles. The first is that good health or poor health is influenced by a set of interrelated factors and requires a multipronged response. The public health model of prevention, wellness, early intervention, and disease management offered good prospects for improved access to care and improved health outcomes.

The second principle subscribes to the notion that when there is community participation in the design, implementation, and evaluation of programs and services, there is greater ownership of the problem and participation in the solution.

The third principle is that effective health care services are not disease-focused but address the whole person. Thus health care agencies are not complete unto themselves; rather, they are part of an interconnected network that offers a broad range of services.

A number of other factors and events contributed to the early development of the model. Recommendations from the conferences pointed to the need to examine how services are organized, used, and delivered in the immigrant's country of origin. It was important to fill this gap because as international migration studies point out (Mason, 1985), Caribbean immigrants strive to maintain strong relationships with their home country in an effort to preserve their cultural identity. They also tend to establish social and support networks and traditional health practices in the new society that closely resemble those to which they are accustomed.

Developing the Model

Building on this contextual framework, several developmental tasks were identified in order to design and develop the Health Keepers Model of service delivery:

- Create a mission statement that reflected CWHA's priorities and was broad enough to allow for growth and flexibility but also narrow enough to maintain focus
- Establish a more formal governance structure, expand the pool of volunteers to advance the mission, and review and amend the by-laws to reflect the mission and structure of the organization
- Strengthen the capacity of CWHA to seek funding and effectively administer grants

Mission
The following mission statement seemed to be most appropriate for CWHA's focus, growth and development: "To provide high-quality, comprehensive, culturally appropriate health, immigration, and social support services to a diverse constituency."

Governance

The existing advisory board was expanded into a formal governance structure that met regulatory requirements, was representative of the population served, and possessed the mix of skills necessary to effectively move the organization forward. In this context, individuals with expertise in community organizing, legal and immigration issues, grant writing and fundraising, public health policy, and program development were sought.

Among the initial activities of the expanded board was the establishment of CWHA's corporate identity. The board created a logo and a slogan ("Strengthening Families and Empowering Communities") and developed a brochure describing the organization's mission, principles, values, programs, and services.

Fund Development

The board began the task of securing grants to broaden the scope of its work to include community outreach, health education, and referral services. The decision to focus its initial efforts on maternal and child health issues stemmed from three factors. First, epidemiological data pointed to disproportionate rates of infant mortality in neighborhoods with a large concentration of Caribbean immigrants compared to the other neighborhoods of Brooklyn and the city of New York. Second, efforts were under way to introduce prenatal care legislation that would grant eligibility for emergency Medicaid for all pregnant women regardless of their immigrant status. And third, funding opportunities for community outreach and education services were among the provisions of the legislation. CWHA was ideally suited to administer this program and submitted a successful application.

Developing Organizational Infrastructure

The theoretical framework for developing CWHA's infrastructure hinged on the work of Kouzes and Mico (1979), who identified policy, management, and service as the three critical domains for decision making and action in human service organizations. It was important that the board of directors and volunteers expeditiously work on all three domains simultaneously in order to fulfill the contractual obligations required by funding sources.

In the policy domain, the board of directors built on its initial work to put in place guidelines for leadership and staff development and policies and procedures for agency management, resource development, and service delivery.

The management domain centered around building leadership and organizational capacity and effectively administering programs in a way that would fulfill CWHA's mission and achieve the following goals:

- Providing outreach and referral mechanisms to increase prenatal care visits for women who would not otherwise access care
- Strengthening families by connecting them with the necessary health, social support, educational, and immigration-related services they need
- Empowering community residents through communitywide action in addressing constituent concerns
- Increasing community collaboration by serving as a link between constituents and mainstream institutions

The service domain revolved around program planning, implementation, and evaluation. It answered questions posed by Kouzes and Mico (1979) relating to the types of services to be provided, how they would be administered to meet the needs of the target population, how CWHA would define the quality of the services provided, and how success would be measured.

Figure 4.1 illustrates the concept and structure for agency startup and implementation of the program using the domain ideas.

Building Organizational Leadership and Capacity

It was clear from all of its prior work that cultural and professional competence would be embodied in all aspects of CWHA functioning. Therefore, a number of competencies to be developed among CWHA's leaders and future employees over time, drawn from existing literature as well as experiential data (Windsor, Baranowski, Clark, and Cutter, 1984), were identified:

- Knowledge of the history, geography, culture, beliefs, practices, and values of the populations to be served

Figure 4.1. CWHA Organizational Structure, 1986.

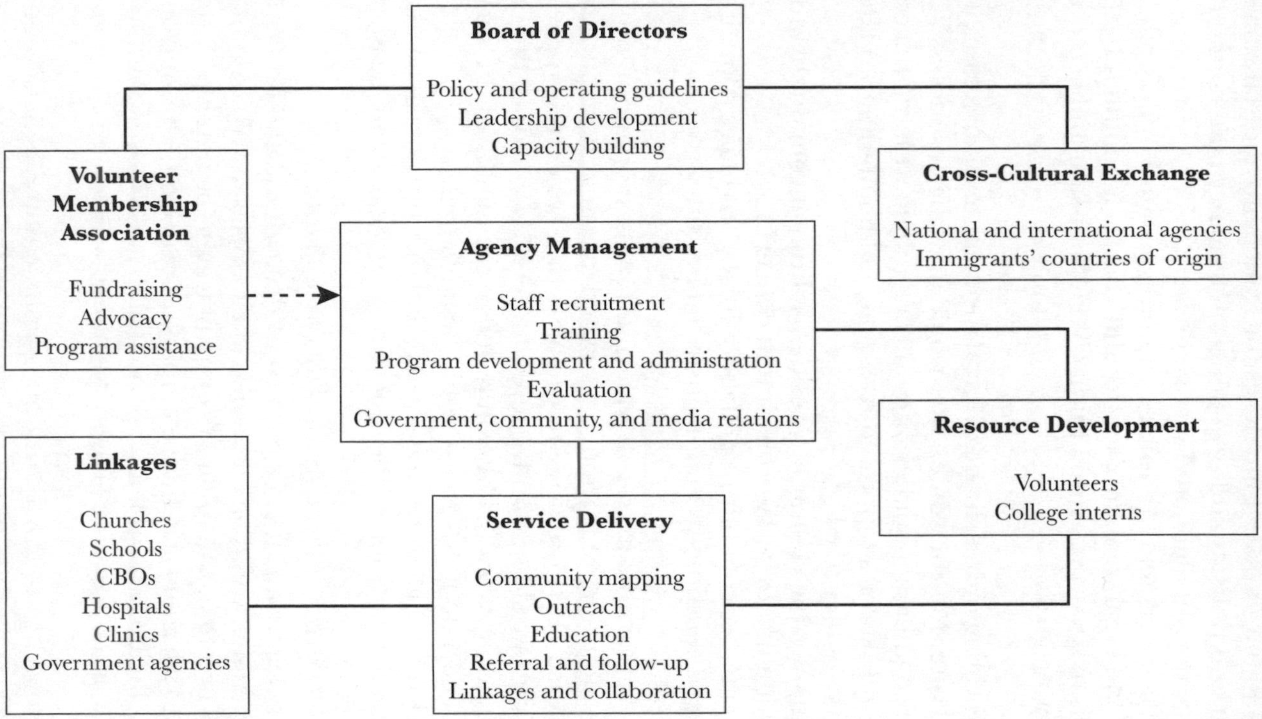

Board of Directors

Policy and operating guidelines
Leadership development
Capacity building

Cross-Cultural Exchange

National and international agencies
Immigrants' countries of origin

Resource Development

Volunteers
College interns

Agency Management

Staff recruitment
Training
Program development and administration
Evaluation
Government, community, and media relations

Volunteer Membership Association

Fundraising
Advocacy
Program assistance

Service Delivery

Community mapping
Outreach
Education
Referral and follow-up
Linkages and collaboration

Linkages

Churches
Schools
CBOs
Hospitals
Clinics
Government agencies

Note: The volunteer membership association is a separate entity that operates like an auxiliary, as indicated by the dotted line.

- Ability to identify the health-related needs of the community and to understand how social, cultural, environmental, and immigration issues affect health behaviors, needs, and interests in that community
- Understanding of the political environment of the community and the history of the relationship between communities, government, and health and social service bureaucracies
- Ability to develop priorities and implement strategies that would enable CWHA to grow
- Ability to obtain community participation in program planning, design, implementation, and evaluation
- Coalition-building skills and ability to foster trust and collaboration between community residents, community-based organizations, and government agencies
- Ability to integrate lessons learned from CWHA's work into an organizational culture that promotes cultural competency

To get the program up and running, employees were recruited and a training curriculum instituted. Figure 4.2 illustrates the components of the training module.

Resource Development

Consumer involvement during this early program planning and implementation stage added the perspective of how services are perceived and used by community residents and what they would like to see done differently.

In addition, involving college interns proved to be a valuable exchange. Internship affords students the opportunity to bridge the gap between theory and practice by participating in community assessment, conference planning, program development and evaluation, and research initiatives. The relationship is equally valuable to CWHA, as students' field study experience and reports are useful for program planning, program enhancement, and evaluation purposes.

Securing volunteers can be extremely challenging in immigrant communities, particularly in situations that require their time and effort during weekdays and traditional working hours. The reason is that in immigrant communities, many individuals have migrated in their adult years and must establish new social and community

Figure 4.2. Training Program for Community Health Workers.

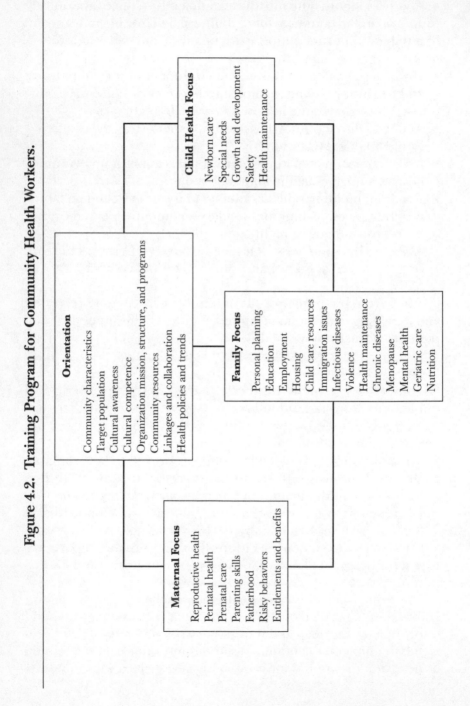

Orientation

Community characteristics
Target population
Cultural awareness
Cultural competence
Organization mission, structure, and programs
Community resources
Linkages and collaboration
Health policies and trends

Child Health Focus

Newborn care
Special needs
Growth and development
Safety
Health maintenance

Maternal Focus

Reproductive health
Perinatal health
Prenatal care
Parenting skills
Fatherhood
Risky behaviors
Entitlements and benefits

Family Focus

Personal planning
Education
Employment
Housing
Child care resources
Immigration issues
Infectious diseases
Violence
Health maintenance
Chronic diseases
Menopause
Mental health
Geriatric care
Nutrition

ties and work long hours to advance professionally and economically. It is also important as immigrant groups become acculturated that they consider recruiting younger volunteers, workers, and organization members, including those born in the United States.

Thus time and financial constraints limit immigrants' ability to volunteer for even the most worthwhile efforts. For those who expressed a willingness to extend themselves, it was important to establish fundamental tenets of participation with which both parties were comfortable. Chief among them were trust and commitment to a shared mission, active participation to accomplish the CWHA's goals and objectives, and a willingness to work together. In return, they were guaranteed efficient functioning in respect of their time, inclusion, and opportunities to be involved in matters relevant to the community.

Implementing the Model

The organizational structure illustrated in Figure 4.1 and the training program in Figure 4.2 provided a framework for service delivery and relationship and capacity building. The following characteristics for effective service delivery were key:

- Employing workers from the community who shared the same cultural and socioeconomic characteristics as the population to be served
- Providing services in English, Spanish, French, and Haitian Creole, the major languages spoken by the target population
- Involving community residents in an advisory capacity in the planning, development, implementation, and evaluation of the program, which proved critical in ensuring that outreach mechanisms, educational curricula, and messages were educationally sound, culturally sensitive, and language-appropriate
- Cultivating relationships with community organizations, faith-based institutions, educational institutions, civic associations, health and human service providers, gatekeepers, community leaders, and elected officials, which helped give acceptance and credibility to program efforts; facilitated client identification, recruitment, and referral; and strengthened advocacy efforts.
- Sharing techniques and best practices with other organizations serving culturally diverse populations

CWHA launched its first government-funded prenatal and education program in 1986. The program was designed to educate the community on the importance and benefits of early and continuous prenatal care and identify and enroll pregnant women in prenatal care.

Gaining community acceptance; engaging the community to become involved in the process; establishing a relationship with the target population, many members of which were undocumented; and assisting them in accessing services were early challenges to be overcome. Several successful strategies were employed.

First and foremost, meetings were held individually with key community leaders and institutions to respond to their concerns about the nature of the program and to enlist their support. Establishing relationships with the target population required approaches that would allay any fear of deportation among the undocumented, clarify issues about entitlement to public benefits, demonstrate sensitivity to the immigrants' linguistic and cultural attributes, and convey a willingness to assist them in maneuvering the health care delivery system.

In addition to popular outreach strategies, such as distribution of flyers and brochures about the program, other strategies used by CWHA to identify and recruit the "hard to reach" included hosting health fairs with churches, civic, health, and community-based organizations; using the ethnic print and electronic media outlets; visiting beauty salons, barbershops, betting establishments, and malls; and setting up tables at street fairs and subway stations.

Establishing rapport with clients, who were often approached while doing their day-to-day business, was a crucial factor in obtaining personal information needed for referral and follow-up. The most significant enabling factor in the engagement process was the personal identification of employees with the language and culture of the client.

Among the early findings of the program were that immigration-related problems served as a major barrier in accessing care and that because of the multitude of issues related to poor birth outcomes, a long-term, family-oriented case management approach would be more effective than a onetime referral for prenatal care.

The first step in being able to provide access to longer-term services for immigrant families was to help those who were undocumented attain legal status and entitlement to benefits and to allay fear among permanent residents and naturalized citizens that using entitlement benefits such as Medicaid and the Women, Infants and Children (WIC) nutrition program would not jeopardize their ability to sponsor relatives. Consequently, in 1987, CWHA established an immigration program to assist undocumented immigrants in adjusting their status under the amnesty provisions of the new immigration law. Over time, the immigration program has expanded in scope and breadth and has become a center of excellence, sharing best practices nationally.

By 1988, CWHA broadened the scope of the prenatal program to include a community health worker perinatal case management component. The main goal of this program was to reduce barriers in accessing perinatal care by coordinating the range of services needed by the pregnant woman and her family. In addition, it provided health education for all women of childbearing age. This program was administered in the adjoining borough of Queens, requiring a new site development for CWHA.

With this expansion came the development of a formalized model of service delivery, the Health Keepers Model (see Figure 4.3), which would be standardized across all of CWHA's existing and future programs regardless of their nature.

Recognizing service gaps in the areas of substance abuse prevention and sickle cell outreach, the community health worker program was expanded in 1992 to include these two areas.

In 1988, by popular demand from community residents, CWHA joined in the struggle to stem the tide of the AIDS epidemic in response to the increasing incidence of the disease throughout New York City, especially in high-risk neighborhoods such as those served by CWHA. The major focus of this education effort, initially, was to heighten community awareness of the disease and its impact on individuals, families, and communities and to offer prevention strategies.

By 1990, it had become evident that culturally sensitive case management services were needed to assist individuals infected with HIV and their families and loved ones, who were affected in turn. This program was further expanded to include a home visitation component intended to promote dialogue among family members and to provide intimate one-on-one education for individuals who had difficulty discussing the issue because of cultural or personal reasons. The program was further expanded to the realm of adolescent HIV education for at-risk youth.

Figure 4.3. The Health Keepers Model.

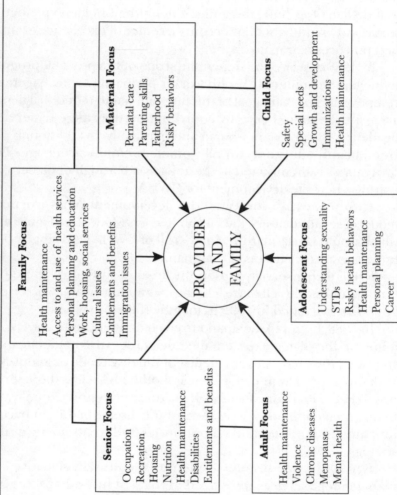

Maternal Focus

Perinatal care
Parenting skills
Fatherhood
Risky behaviors

Child Focus

Safety
Special needs
Growth and development
Immunizations
Health maintenance

Family Focus

Health maintenance
Access to and use of health services
Personal planning and education
Work, housing, social services
Cultural issues
Entitlements and benefits
Immigration issues

Adolescent Focus

Understanding sexuality
STDs
Risky health behaviors
Health maintenance
Personal planning
Career

Senior Focus

Occupation
Recreation
Housing
Nutrition
Health maintenance
Disabilities
Entitlements and benefits

Adult Focus

Health maintenance
Violence
Chronic diseases
Menopause
Mental health

PROVIDER AND FAMILY

As word of the effectiveness of CWHA's service delivery model spread, CWHA was provided with funding in 1992 to conduct a needs assessment of Caribbean immigrants with developmental disabilities. Subsequently, a resource manual for providers was developed and published.

By 1996, CWHA had established two additional sites, one as an expansion of the community health worker perinatal program in a different area of the borough of Queens and a WIC nutrition program to provide vouchers and nutrition education to pregnant women and children.

As Medicaid Managed Care came into being, CWHA also contracted with managed care organizations to provide consumer education on the managed care system, its benefits, their rights as consumers, and how to choose a plan.

In 1997, CWHA introduced its domestic violence prevention and case management initiative in collaboration with the Brooklyn district attorney's office, as its target area had the highest number of reports of domestic violence in the borough. Also in 1997, CWHA contracted with the Greater New York March of Dimes to provide intensive perinatal case management to high-risk women, operating from a local hospital.

As CWHA broadened its services, it became clear that it would be wise to use the same service delivery model to provide primary care services. CWHA therefore entered into partnership with a local hospital in 1998 and established the Caribbean-American Family Health Center, with a capacity to handle ten thousand annual primary care visits. The hospital provided clinical services, while CWHA concentrated on its centers of excellence, outreach and referrals, education, case management, and immigration services.

Since 1998, CWHA has focused on maintaining its complement of services while contracting with foundations and other institutions to implement short-term research and education projects in the areas of breast health and cancer research and screening. By 2003, CWHA had built a network of services as illustrated in Figure 4.4.

Successes

In its two decades of existence, CWHA has matured into a service agency with a portfolio of accomplished projects and expertise in meeting the health, immigration, and social support needs of immigrants and the poor. That expertise represents an aggressive commitment to CWHA's core principles of strengthening families, empowering communities, and building bridges across diverse cultures. The organization has grown from a group of twelve volunteers to five fully staffed community service centers, providing services to thousands of families annually.

CWHA's successes are demonstrated each and every day as pregnant women are prepared with skills and services for childbearing and child rearing, adolescents are taught skills that strengthen their self-esteem, HIV-infected individuals and their families receive the support they need, individuals without food and shelter are assisted to secure those basic necessities, immigrants are aided in adjusting to the mainstream of American life, and healthy lifestyles for all are promoted.

Figure 4.4. Organization of CWHA Services, 2003.

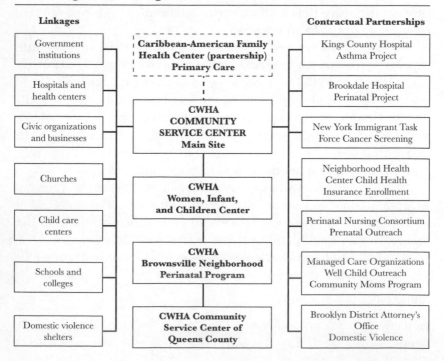

As community members use the health and social services offered, they look to CWHA as a concerned and trusted friend of the community. Integral to the success are strong public, private sector, and community partnerships shaped into a service network. Since CWHA's inception, establishing formal and informal linkages has played an important role in client recruitment, referral, case management, and service delivery. Collaborations and partnerships exist too for information sharing, benchmarking, and promotion of best practices and resource development. Others are formed for cooperative purchasing and funding opportunities, and others, such as those with United Way of New York City and the Federation of Protestant Welfare Agencies, for technical assistance, resource building, and funding opportunities.

These partnerships, together with effective leadership, a committed and dedicated board of directors and employees, and community involvement and accountability, have created a powerful synergy that has sustained CWHA's growth.

Many lessons have been learned over the course of CWHA's two decades of community service, but the three elements most responsible for the organization's success are these:

• When health care providers and systems listen to their patients and the communities they serve, better health outcomes are the lasting result.
• Leadership from trusted and credible neighborhood-based organizations is an essential element for planning, partnering, and delivering services in poor and culturally diverse communities.
• Any attempt to address the health care needs of underserved populations must include providing families with economic opportunities, social networks, and services that help them find and remain in decent and affordable housing, keep their children in school and help them succeed, obtain jobs that pay a living wage, provide a career path, secure health and social services, build assets and create wealth, and contribute to the revitalization of their neighborhoods.

In terms of quantity of services delivered, on the local neighborhood level, CWHA has an impressive record of accomplishment in its various program areas. In 1986, the prenatal program served two thousand pregnant women with a budget of $82,000, one program manager, and four part-time staff. In contrast, by 2004, the budget had grown to $3.5 million, with forty-five full-time employees serving over thirty thousand individuals through outreach, education, case management, and direct services.

CWHA's excellence in service delivery has been widely acclaimed for its quality, breadth, and impact. In 2000, CWHA received the New York State Department of Health's Health Education Award, and the following year the department's award for Excellence in Public Health.

On the national front, CWHA has become a respected institution for its service delivery to culturally diverse populations. The organization has been sought out to share its best practices in strategic partnership building, service delivery modalities, and organizational development with small organizations nationwide.

Internationally, CWHA is accredited as a nongovernmental organization (NGO) by the United Nations Economic and Social Council. CWHA has participated in public health activities in the circum-Caribbean region, Latin America, Europe, Egypt, South Africa, and Asia.

In evaluating the strengths of CWHA, the following were drawn from an organizational needs assessment by consultants from the National Executive Service Corps (Wheeler, 1998):

- A very strong sense of vision is widely evidenced. CWHA is attuned to the unique cultural needs of the agency's client population and how these people are affected by environmental changes.
- CWHA enjoys a unique reputation of providing the highest level of commitment and service to its clients, and CWHA enjoys the respect and confidence of the people in the community it serves.
- The organization is knowledgeable about the community it serves and is very aggressive in pursuing its mission.
- A high degree of personal commitment by staff is evidenced, and there is great willingness to work hard and to work long hours.
- Based on feedback from surveys received from clients, CWHA delivers services in a very competent manner. A good process

for measuring client satisfaction is employed in the majority of the agency's activities.

- Self-expectations are well communicated through program write-ups and position descriptions.
- Accessibility to senior staff is very good.
- Planning skills are well demonstrated on a project or programmatic level where the need for many trade-off decisions is limited.
- Ability to deliver services is well documented.
- Political and economic ties are well established.
- Ability to work creatively within the system and withstand bureaucratic pressures has been well demonstrated.
- Linkages with primary care providers are well established.

Challenges

In a very short period of time, CWHA has emerged as a leading organization with a grassroots response in effectively addressing the multiple and complex needs of a large segment of New York City's expanding Caribbean immigrant community.

The organization's advocacy and service delivery mechanism has been embraced by government and other funders and viewed as an opportunity to improve access to and delivery of health care to underserved communities. Therefore, CWHA was able to access government money to address the most pressing problems affecting its constituents.

The rapid development of CWHA and increasing demand for services left little time for planning to ensure the organization's long-term sustainability. CWHA is overly dependent on government contracts. This means that approximately 80 percent of its revenues come from government, and those monies are largely limited to supporting service delivery with little available for administrative services and infrastructure building. As a result, CWHA has continuously grappled with an increasingly weak infrastructure.

Early on, CWHA recognized that overreliance on erratic government funding streams was problematic. Over the period 1989–1992, a fund balance deficit and an almost perpetual cash flow problem affected the agency's ability to make timely payments on payroll and operating expenses.

Because of this experience, it became apparent that CWHA must not only decrease its dependency on government funding but also renegotiate the terms under which it will accept government funds. Consequently, government funds were no longer accepted in amounts that were insufficient to carry the full operating expense of a particular program, including allocated overhead. Further, no spending occurred until CWHA signed a contract that held the funding source liable for monies spent. The payoff for these strategies came in 1993, when CWHA had an increase in fund balance after meeting all expenses at the end of the fiscal year.

In addition, CWHA made concerted efforts to secure nongovernmental funds by cultivating relationships with foundations and corporations, maximizing the fundraising efforts of its volunteer membership auxiliary through special events, and expanding immigration services to include a fee-for-service component. Again these strategies paid off. For example, private grants and other income increased by 259 percent from 1990 to 1993, while government funding rose only 3 percent over the same period.

Unfortunately, this trend did not continue. Efforts to raise money from private sources, through special events, and from fee-for-service immigration activities presented formidable challenges for a variety of reasons.

During the 1990s, private foundations and corporations began to tie their funding to service outcomes, widening the gap for administrative and other than personnel services normally filled by these grants. New immigration policies and practices created fewer opportunities for special programs available to immigrants from the Caribbean, and ancillary services such as fingerprinting offered by CWHA organizations for a fee were disallowed by the Immigration and Naturalization Service. A major portion of this income was previously used to fill needed gaps not covered by grants, such as consultant fees, enhancing technology, and other capacity-building efforts.

In addition, CWHA's board of directors, like many nonprofit boards, was limited in its ability to raise the unrestricted funds necessary to reduce the increasing cash flow problems created by government contracts.

Further, in an increasingly financially restrictive health care environment, government contracts have become flat despite the rising cost of operating programs. This has left little for administrative and other than personnel services, further weakening the organization's infrastructure.

The major weaknesses revolve around the following matters:

- The organization is very thin at the administrative levels, with few personnel who can serve as backstops ready to move up to positions of higher authority.
- There is a lack of secretarial support as well as administrative support to enable the executive director and the heads of finance and personnel to devote time to long-range issues rather than those of a day-to-day nature.
- The level of planning for the total organization is limited to planning for specific programs with very little time for long-term forecasting.
- The organization's board of directors is not a major contributor in ways that successful nonprofit boards usually are, and CWHA had never had a board of directors strong enough to enable it to carry out the plans it wished to undertake and the range of fundraising activities necessary to support those plans.
- Fundraising is not one of the organization's strengths other than through the granting process for programs.
- A low overhead allowance in government grants and the fact that funds are reimbursed only after expenses are incurred are the primary factors causing CWHA's cash flow deficit.
- CWHA has no endowment or other financial cushion to enable it to cope with erratic cash flows endemic to government-funded programs.
- Shrinking grant dollars and constant demand for services have forced programs to be underfunded, and the grant process allowed little or no flexibility in redirecting budget items to better carry out program objectives.
- Resources are limited.
- The organization is at times forced to cut back services in the face of increased demand for help.

Future Outlook

It is clear that to address its current problems, needs, opportunities, and challenges, CWHA needs to reflect on its past growth and plan for future development while maintaining the quality of its services and its stability. First and foremost is the need to plan strategically. The following must be key components of the strategic plan:

- An internal analysis of CWHA's mission, history, financial performance, strengths, weaknesses, and market position. The profile should conclude with an identification of critical issues facing CWHA that will serve as a framework for developing strategic initiatives.
- A service area analysis to examine the population currently served by CWHA and the population it intends to serve in the future. Specifics of this profile should include demographic, socioeconomic, and health indicators and cultural characteristics within those communities; the sociopolitical environment; and market forces. Trends in funding and gaps in services delivery should also be examined.
- Redefinition of the mission, goals, and priorities of the organization to reflect its current and future position.
- Development of a set of strategies to enable CWHA to address its current and future opportunities and challenges.

Conclusion

Despite its growth and success over the years, many challenges remain. Like other nonprofits, CWHA has sharpened its efforts to attract funding to provide services in the areas of highest need for the ethnic and immigrant communities of New York City. CWHA continues to move forward with a strong commitment to service and to meeting community needs. At the same time, the organization has redoubled its efforts at achieving financial independence as a critical step toward long-term sustainability.

In pursuit of these two goals, CWHA has conducted strategic planning with the help of United Way and other agencies that provide technical assistance to nonprofits. Current activities include efforts to decrease dependency on government grants and to broaden its base of support. In that regard, CWHA has embarked on an effort to increase board size and to diversify board composition. The intent is to continue meeting the challenges that are ahead through careful planning and preparation.

Key Points

- This comprehensive case study of CWHA traced the development and operation of a CBHO and its service delivery model specifically designed to respond to the health needs of ethnic and immigrant groups in New York City.
- The historical account of CWHA's origins and growth provided evidence of the need for health to be defined from a community perspective, the importance of understanding the beliefs and practices of the population being served, and the effectiveness of delivering health services to ethnic and immigrant groups from a neighborhood-based, integrated, and comprehensive perspective.
- CWHA's success is due in part to the fact that its founding members, as residents of the communities being served, understood the need to address health care issues as part of the larger socioeconomic concerns of poor families, which includes the multiple dimensions of affordable and safe housing, economic opportunities, functioning schools, and living wages.
- The Health Keepers Model is grounded in the understanding that health outcomes are the product of interrelated factors and that effective health service delivery therefore requires multipronged inputs and coordinated responses.
- In two decades, CWHA has matured into a service agency with a track record of accomplished projects and expertise in health, immigration, and social support services to immigrants and the poor.
- CWHA started with a group of twelve volunteers and currently has five fully staffed community service centers providing services to thousands of families annually.
- Despite challenges, careful strategic planning will keep the future outlook positive.

Study Questions

1. Select any large metropolitan area in the United States. You have just been hired as a health provider at a local hospital in this city. The hospital serves distinct population groups plagued by long-term health disparities. In preparation for this new job, you must

draft a brief paper for your new employers in which you outline your approach for providing prevention education services to residents of the local neighborhood surrounding the hospital who also experience poor health outcomes. In the paper, you will report on the health indicators for that group, including socioeconomic levels and numbers of uninsured individuals. Then, carefully investigate and document all information on the members of that group that you can find regarding their history, socioeconomic condition, religion, family system and roles, health beliefs and practices, and legal and immigration issues.

2. Describe the community in which you reside in terms of its demographic makeup, rates of health insurance, socioeconomic levels and health indicators, health beliefs and practices, family systems and roles, and sources of health information. Based on this information, answer the following questions: What barriers to health care exist in your community, and what agencies operate to help residents overcome those barriers? What are the critical gaps in service delivery? How do you propose to fill those gaps?

References

"Achievements in Public Health, 1900–1999: Healthier Mothers and Babies." *Morbidity and Mortality Weekly Report,* 1999, *48,* 849–858.

Antoine, L. B. "Mental Health Care, Cultural Beliefs, and Compatibility of Health Services in the Caribbean." Paper presented at the Caribbean Women's Health Association conference Delivering Culturally Compatible Health Care to Immigrants, New York, Oct. 1985.

Bogen, E. *Caribbean Immigrants in New York City: A Demographic Summary.* New York: New York City Department of City Planning, Office of Immigrant Affairs, 1985.

Browne, R, Graham, Y. J., and Hylton, D. (eds.). *Delivering Culturally Compatible Perinatal Care Services to Immigrants: The Caribbean Population in New York City.* New York: Caribbean Women's Health Association, 1986.

Center for New York City Affairs, Robert J. Milano Graduate School of Management and Urban Policy, New School University. *Consider the Future: Strengthening Children and Family Services in Red Hook.* New York: Center for New York City Affairs, 2003.

Chavkin, W. "Epidemiological Perspective of Reproductive Health of Caribbean Women in New York City." Paper presented at the Caribbean Women's Health Association conference Delivering Culturally Compatible Health Care to Immigrants, New York, Oct. 1985.

Frank, H. "Voodoo, Santeria, and Folk Health Practices." Paper presented at the Caribbean Women's Health Association conference Delivering Culturally Compatible Health Care to Immigrants, New York, Oct. 1985.

Frank, H. "Understanding Haitian Religious Beliefs, Cultural Issues, Challenges, and Barriers to Acceptance of Conventional HIV/AIDS Care." Paper presented at the Health Conference on AIDS in the Caribbean-American Community, New York, Dec. 7, 2001.

Freiden, T. R. *Infant Mortality in New York City: Trends and Strategies.* New York: Department of Health and Mental Hygiene, 2002.

Freire, P. *Pedagogy of the Oppressed.* New York: Continuum, 1990.

Fruchter, R., Boyce, J., and Hunt, M. "Missed Opportunities for Early Diagnosis of Cancer of the Cervix." *American Journal of Public Health,* 1980, *70,* 418–420.

Heckler, M. M. *Report of the Secretary's Task Force on Black and Minority Health,* Vol. 2: *Crosscutting Issues in Minority Health.* Washington, D.C.: U.S. Department of Health and Human Services, 1985.

Kleinman, A., Eisenberg, L., and Good, B. "Culture, Illness and Care." *Annals of Internal Medicine,* 1978, *88,* 251–258.

Kouzes, J. M., and Mico, P. R. "Domain Theory: An Introduction to Organizational Behavior in Human Service Organizations." *Journal of Applied Behavioral Science,* 1979, *19,* 449–469.

Leicher, S. *Voices from the Field—Building Bridges and Removing Barriers: A Strategy to Promote the Self-Sufficiency of New York's Immigrant Communities.* New York: United Way, 2001.

Malone, T. E., and Johnson, K. W. *Report of the Secretary's Task Force on Black and Minority Health,* Vol. 6: *Infant Mortality and Low Birthweight.* Washington, D.C.: U.S. Department of Health and Human Services, 1986.

Mason, M. A. "The Development of a Framework for Health Care Advocacy on Behalf of Caribbean Immigrants: Causal Scheme of Poor Health Among Migrants." Doctoral dissertation. University Microfilms International, Ann Arbor, Mich., 1985.

McKnight, J. L., and Kretzmann, J. P. "Mapping Community Capacity." In M. Minkler (ed.), *Community and Community Building for Health.* New Brunswick, N.J.: Rutgers University Press, 2002.

McLaughlin, M. "Cultural and Linguistics Barriers: A Reality for English-Speaking Immigrants." Paper presented at the Caribbean Women's Health Association conference Delivering Culturally Compatible Health Care to Immigrants, New York, Oct. 1985.

Mintz, S. W. *Caribbean Transformations.* Hawthorne, N.Y.: Aldine de Gruyter, 1974.

New York City Department of City Planning. *NYC 2000: Results from the 2000 Census.* New York: Department of City Planning, 2002.

New York State Public Health Council. *Communities Working Together for a Healthier New York: Opportunities to Improve the Health of New Yorkers*. Albany: New York State Public Health Council, 1996.

Office of the District Attorney, Kings County (Brooklyn), New York. *Violence Against Women (VAWA) Project Report*. Brooklyn, N.Y.: Office of the District Attorney, 2002.

Siska, D. *Responding to Immigrant Needs: Before and After September 11*. New York: New York Regional Association of Grantmakers, 2002.

Thomas, B. J. "Caribbean Voluntary Associations and the Development of Brooklyn." In *The New Muse Community Museum of Brooklyn: An Introduction to the Black Contribution to the Development of Brooklyn*. Brooklyn, N.Y.: New Muse Community Museum of Brooklyn, 1977.

U.S. Census Bureau. "Ancestry: Census 2000 Supplementary Survey." [http://www.census.gov/population/www/ancestry.html]. 2003.

Wheeler, I. Strategic plan developed for the Caribbean Women's Health Association. New York: National Executive Service Corps, 1998.

Windsor, R. A., Baranowski, T., Clark, N. M., and Cutter, G. *Evaluation of Health Promotion and Education Programs*. Mountain View, Calif.: Mayfield, 1984.

The CBHO Environment and Models for the Future

The three chapters in Part Three are vital to understanding the ongoing operations and future of CBHOs. Chapter Five's focus is on the political and economic environment of CBHOs and how that environment influences management activities. CBHOs are being called on to increase their skill level so as not only to provide services but also to engage in advocating for resources and policy changes.

Chapter Six reports on the lessons learned, pitfalls, and best practices of surviving CBHOs. It provides a framework that serves to guide the growth and development of organizational capacity building, without which long-term sustainability of CBHOs is difficult to achieve. Step-by-step guidance is provided for developing and implementing the full range of organizational structures and operating tools, from mission and vision to strategic planning and staffing.

U.S. health services in their present form are a hodgepodge of funding streams, a potpourri of plans, an outdated medical model that continues to influence medical training and service delivery, and persistent health disparities that can and must be eliminated. Chapter Seven focuses on projections regarding the creation of a health care system in the United States that will be able to deliver health care for all, based on an analysis of international and national efforts to provide health care services to diverse populations.

Chapter Five

The Political and Economic Management of CBHOs

Marcia Bayne Smith

In the 1970s, the federal government began to systematically transfer to local and state governments responsibility for providing services to their residents. Following the federal trend, state and city governments subsequently engaged in a similar transfer of responsibility, initially for social services, increasingly for health, and most recently for educational services, onto the shoulders of the nonprofit sector. The burden of that transfer has forced community-based organizations (CBOs) and community-based health organizations (CBHOs) to engage in unprecedented political maneuvering as a matter of survival. Further, CBHOs must now develop multiple skill sets beyond what is required for service delivery that will also enable them to serve as focal points for organizing and mobilizing their communities to advocate for improved health outcomes.

Learning Objectives

- State legislatures determine how much power city governments have and the services they must provide for citizens.
- In the 1970s and 1980s, the federal government instituted a policy that became known as the "devolution revolution." Devolution is the practice of transferring responsibility for providing services to citizens from local state and city governments.

The theory behind devolution is that local government can provide local services better than the federal government.

- Local governments subsequently followed suit and transferred to the nonprofit sector responsibility for the delivery of social services, especially in the areas of health, child welfare, family services, and in some cases education-related services. This transfer from local government to nonprofits was more difficult, as it was done with diminished resources, increased demands for greater levels of services, and almost no technical assistance to the nonprofits in taking on these new responsibilities.

- To survive, nonprofits have had to develop a mix of skills that equip them to negotiate for their share of city resources.

- Community groups must resist the psychological manipulation of zero-sum thinking.

- Developing cross-organizational collaborations that pull resources and energies together is a political strategy that forces decision makers to increase the size of the resource pie instead of continually shrinking it.

- Advocacy has become an indispensable skill to CBHO survival.

- CBHOs that engage in political advocacy can extract necessary goods and services from the system and contribute to long-term community sustainability.

The Political and Economic Environment of CBHOs

CBHOs and the communities they serve are part of the larger political and economic framework of local government structures. In that regard, the resources available at the local level, whether urban or rural, as well as the decision-making systems that are used in each local area to determine how resources are distributed, all affect the ability of a CBHO to operate. We shall briefly assess political and economic functioning at the local level with a focus on cities and then examine the political and economic relationship between cities and the nonprofit sector, specifically community-based organizations.

Two sets of structural constraints affect the management of cities. One has to do with the way government is politically organized in the United States, and the other has to do with capitalism and its impact on local economies. The caveat here is that although we will discuss political and economic structures separately, they are inextricably intertwined, and any mention of the one has implications for the other.

According to the Constitution of the United States, legal and political power to enact and implement policy is concentrated at the federal and state levels of government. This is understandable because when the Constitution was adopted in 1789, cities were few and small, and founders of the Republic saw no need to grant them any extensive self-governing powers. However, by 1865, after the Civil War, industrialization and immigration fueled the expansion of cities. As cities grew, they became politically, economically, and socially so difficult to manage that by the nineteenth century, the states eventually opted to grant cities the right, with limitations, to govern themselves.

Up to that point, most U.S. cities had been governed by volunteer members of the upper classes. By the 1800s, cities opted to be governed by a city council that was elected to office. The U.S. Constitution provides guarantees of "one man, one vote," and so the working-class voters easily elected the majority of the members of the city councils in most cities because the working class far outnumbered the upper classes. As city council members became more powerful, they frequently accepted bribes in exchange for some city services or favors.

The upper classes, primarily wealthy business owners, soon grew tired of paying bribes to conduct business. As businessmen, they were well aware that the U.S. Constitution, like the constitutions of other nations, is both a political and an economic document. The founders, intent on building a prosperous nation, made certain that the Constitution carefully described the critical provisions of a free-market economy. For example, Article 1, section 8, gives Congress the right to regulate commerce among the states, with foreign nations, and with the sovereign Indian tribes. It also gives Congress the power to coin money and punish counterfeiting, and section 10 gives that power exclusively to Congress by indicating that "no state shall have the right . . . to coin money." The U.S. Constitution is unquestionably a very thorough economic document that covers the breadth of economic enterprise, including contracts, copyrights, exports, searches and seizures, and due process.

Mindful that as members of the business class they possessed full constitutional backing, the upper classes set out to wrest control of city government from the working classes. First they organized themselves into a powerful group. Then they accused city councils of corruption, and next they put political pressure on state governments to change the city council system. As can be expected, the result was acquiescence at the state level, which transformed city politics in two critical ways, described in the following section, and have lasted until today.

Managing Cities: The Political and Economic Issues

First, the decision-making power to run cities was assigned to city mayors or city managers in some states. Second and probably more important, along with mayors came political machines, which are formidable vehicles for corruption. Political machines are highly organized structures that centralize power in a political boss. At the same time, they are also capable of satisfying the needs of diverse subgroups and individuals in the larger community by providing tangible rewards that are not usually available through legal or culturally approved means (Merton, 1957). Today, political machines no longer function as overtly as they once did. For example, political machines were credited with getting voters to the polls in record numbers in the past. Nevertheless, machines are still around, and they still wield considerable influence, as borne out by the case of a Democratic Party boss of a New York City borough who was recently accused of maintaining the century-old process of controlling the appointment of judges from Brooklyn to the state supreme court, despite efforts to reform that old boys' network (Eaton, 2003).

State governments granted cities the right to self-rule, but with several limitations. These limitations were intended, on the one hand, to force local government to provide needed services to city residents. On the other hand, recognizing the political pressure they had already endured because of city politics, state governments sought to break up the control that local political machines had over city government. These were good intentions; however, state governments have not eased the limitations on city government in more than a century, and this limited authority of city governments has had two major sorts of impacts.

One major impact of these limitations is that they gave rise to a new kind of politics in which managers of cities must be mindful of the demands of state government but in large metropolitan areas cities must also compete, much more so now in a globalized economy, with other cities in their perceived "market" to attract large corporations and jobs. Thus these limitations place cities at the mercy of the formal business community and its corporations. Cities are forced to give in to corporate demands for tax abatements, subsidies, and other benefits because cities do not want to lose business and jobs to a competitor city.

The result is that today, cities across the nation rely primarily on property taxes for revenue, with smaller income from business taxes and much smaller income from service fees for items such as water and garbage collection, which are just a small part of the range of services that cities provide to residents. Only a small number of cities are able to generate additional revenue through tourism. At one point in time, cities were able to increase their tax base by annexing surrounding areas or by increasing their population through immigration. These methods no longer work because in most cities, especially in the Northeast, any annexation effort would be met with fierce resistance. Furthermore, although the immigration reforms of the past two decades have not totally stopped immigrant flows into U.S. cities, those policy changes served to curtail the influx of new taxpayers. Therefore, cities have become more dependent on state governments for funding, due to their limited ability to generate new revenues to pay for the ever-increasing cost of services they are mandated by the state to provide (Shannon, Kleniewski, and Cross, 1997).

The other large impact of state limitations on cities can be found in the informal political structure. In the formal system, votes are cast for a candidate for office, and the candidate with the most votes wins. Separate from this legal system is a whole other informal political system in which powerful people, who have not been elected to a political office, have the power to influence policy decisions and outcomes in their own favor. This informal political structure consists of individuals and groups of people who are often, but not always, wealthy. In addition to owners of businesses, the informal political system includes unions and professionals and their professional organizations (for example, doctors and the American Medical Association and hospitals, their executives, and the American

Hospital Association). Also wielding substantial political power and influence are organized interest groups and individuals involved in social movements such as gay rights and religious organizations.

These various groups exert influence on the formal political system through a variety of means, from large monetary contributions to the political campaigns of elected officials to the effective use of media and manipulation of public opinion.

Thus cities are challenging areas to manage because of their limited power to self-govern, competition between cities to raise revenues from a finite set of sources such as tourism, the constantly increasing list of state-imposed services that must be provided to city residents and the nature of those services, limits on the type and amount of taxes that can be collected at the city level, and the constant pressure from the informal political system.

Managing Cities: Searching for Political and Economic Balance

In an effort to manage cities properly and remain in office, city officials develop finely tuned skills for negotiation, collaboration, and on occasion the ability to take a stand. On the one hand, city officials are bombarded by requests from businesses that must be handled well for several reasons. First, improved business profits can mean keeping existing businesses in the city and attracting new ones. More important for elected officials, businesses are the largest contributors to political campaigns and so are not to be alienated. On the other hand, facing constant political pressure from organized community groups, concerned citizens, and other interest groups all wanting to have their needs met, city officials must strike a balance among all these demands. However, some critics say there is no contest because the two major responsibilities of cities are to provide every opportunity for businesses to operate and to prevent any effort to overthrow the economic system.

The political and economic problems of cities across the United States are exacerbated by the fact that politics and economics are inextricably intertwined. Cities started out as colonial villages and remained that way for more than two hundred years, during which time the national economy was primarily agricultural. Urban areas began to grow in the 1800s, especially after the Civil War, and continued to do so through the mid-1900s as a result of industrialization and immigration, becoming large metropolitan centers of commerce. After World War II, cities contracted and withered economically largely because federal policy provided fiscal incentives to the states for the building of highways, financial subsidies to developers to build suburban residential and business areas, and federally backed mortgages, all of which encouraged people and businesses to move out to the suburbs. The contraction of cities that started in the 1950s sent the inner core of cities into a spiraling decline of joblessness, substandard housing and schooling, racial segregation, and poor health that reached its peak in the 1980s. Economic changes continue today to assail the stability of cities.

The Information Revolution and the new service economy it spawned helped some cities remain afloat by creating a few jobs at the high end of the economic spectrum, along with many more low-income jobs. In the 1990s, new urban policies were developed, such as the Federal HOPE VI program, which provides monies to replace public housing, and state programs to develop "economic enterprise zones." The concern is that programs such as HOPE VI contribute to gentrification and economic enterprise zones are designed to help business owners; neither of them results in benefits for poor inner-city residents and communities. For the most part, however, cities continue to face shrinking support from federal and state government as well as an ever-widening income gap, both of which contribute to health disparities among the poorest segments of the population.

City Governance and Health Care Services

The governance of cities requires that city officials engage in a constant balancing of political and economic realities. Elected officials must pit their political goals and ambitions against the relentless efforts of interest groups, particularly wealthy business owners, to obtain tax concessions and other savings from city coffers while not losing sight of the responsibility to provide services to everyone living in the city. And therein lies the dilemma: in cities, there is a distinct difference in the quality of services provided to poor and working-class residents and those available to the wealthy. Health care services are a perfect example. In wealthy areas, private physicians' offices abound, the numbers of residents with private insurance is high, and the health needs of the wealthy are usually well met. This is not the case in poor or working-class neighborhoods.

Although large municipal and voluntary hospitals exist in poor neighborhoods, and despite the use of the emergency rooms of these hospitals for routine care, they do not constitute a "medical home" or source of regular ongoing medical care with a consistent provider, both of which are major contributors to good health. Further, as city coffers are stretched to support the municipals, there is very little support for health education that would teach city residents, especially poor residents, about the benefits of practicing preventive medicine and obtaining care from a steady source.

Therefore, it is in poor and some working-class communities that CBHOs are likely to be established, as they are traditionally the health care providers in underserved areas. In the process of establishing CBHOs, community groups learn to become advocates and to function as other interest groups do in terms of the pressure they must place on elected officials. However, unlike interest groups such as corporations or unions, CBHOs and the communities they serve are significantly more adversely affected by changes in federal policy such as devolution.

The Federal Government's Role in City Health Services

From the Johnson administration through the Carter administration, the health care issues that city governments dealt with included the perceived lack of primary care physicians located in poor neighborhoods, the limited number of practitioners willing to accept poor or uninsured patients, how best to address the episodic nature of hospital-based outpatient departments and emergency rooms, and how to respond to the fallout that would result if the government were to establish ambulatory care provider services within proximity of public or voluntary hospitals, which would be interpreted as a deliberate attack on the revenues of those institutions.

Although it is clear in hindsight that early resolution of these issues would have been less expensive thirty years ago, cost was nevertheless a serious issue in the depressed economy of the 1970s. At that time, the concerns around cost included availability of third-party payers, allowable Medicare and Medicaid reimbursements, the restrictions placed on income from grants for public health clinics, and the need to bill and collect for services even from poor patients who traditionally received services for free.

The ability of local governments to provide health and mental health services for the poor worsened throughout the 1970s and even more in the 1980s. Largely to blame were four distinct economic and sociopolitical phenomena that occurred in the two decades between 1965 and 1985. First, cities lost significant portions of their tax base due to the migration of upper-income people to the suburbs, leaving behind in the inner cities a concentration of people with middle to lower incomes. Second, the transformation of the U.S. economy from a manufacturing base to a globalized, high-tech information society that had been under way since the end of World War II was now being felt, especially by those left behind in the cities. Third, immigration laws from the 1960s in preparation for the new service economy allowed an influx of primarily poor and low-skilled immigrants. Finally, with the arrival of the Reagan administration in Washington in 1981, government stepped back from social spending at the city level.

The Devolution Revolution

The early urban policies of the 1950s and 1960s, particularly the programs of the Johnson administration's "Great Society," provided and administered federal dollars to fund programs in the inner city. This created a problem because federal control over city programs not only made cities dependent on federal funds in order to provide services to their residents but also threw cities into fiscal crisis whenever cuts in federal funding were made. To reverse this dependency and stabilize the situation, the federal government instituted a policy, beginning in the 1970s, that would later become know as the "devolution revolution."

Devolution is defined as "passing policy responsibilities from the federal government to state governments in the form of block grants, reduced grants-in-aid, and increased state flexibility to comply with federal mandates. The intent of devolution is to improve federal government efficiency based on the theory that local government can do a better job of providing services to citizens" (Conservation

Company, 2000, p. C-1). Devolution allows the federal government to transfer the responsibility for providing services to citizens to local (state and city) governments. The problem is that at the same time that the federal government made devolution the preferred method for sharing responsibility for citizen services with local governments, it simultaneously cut back on the amount of money provided to the states to pay for those services (Watson and Gold, 1997).

The combination of devolution decisions by government and globalization decisions by corporations has had deleterious effects on the health, economy, and general well-being of many local communities, both urban and rural. Part of the problem is that since the 1990s, state and local city governments have followed the federal lead and are now passing on to local community-based agencies the responsibility of providing services to local residents without adequate economic support. The result is city governments, CBOs, and CBHOs struggling under the weight of this new burden.

For example, Medicaid is public health insurance for people who are poor, permanently disabled, pregnant, blind, elderly, or mothers with dependent children. Medicaid was one of the programs that the Reagan administration included in its devolution policy in the 1980s by providing states with a "block grant" for Medicaid. Block grants are a lump sum of money that the federal government sends to the states and cities to be used in specified but loosely interpreted ways. This means, for example, that a block grant for education would take the place of individual targeted funding for art education programs or music programs in city schools. Instead of the federal government establishing these programs and providing funds for them, the national government simply provides a pot of money for education, and it is then up to the states and cities to determine how best to spend it and on what programs. The problem here is that the states are not always committed to use all of their education money for education programs.

In providing a block grant to the states to administer Medicaid, the federal government accomplished two objectives in the 1980s. The responsibility for providing health care to poor people was effectively transferred to the states and cities, and the grants to the states for providing this service were for less money than the federal government had been spending to run the program. States and cities had no alternative but to cut services to their citizens.

Health Policies of the 1980s and 1990s and Their Impact on Community Health

Three fundamental shifts in health policy and resources occurred during the Reagan years that have had the greatest impact on the health of poor and working-class communities. The first of these, as previously discussed, involved policy decisions to reduce overall health and social spending through the use of block grants and other policy devices. In the health arena in particular, this translated into reductions in state-level Medicaid spending, underfinancing of community health centers, and decreased municipal subsidies for free medical care. As a result, more and more people in inner-city neighborhoods came to depend on public hospitals and hospital emergency rooms for their health care. At the same time, the amount and quality of care that public hospitals and community health centers could provide decreased (Dutton, 1987).

A second policy shift, which started in the 1970s, was also taking shape in the 1980s while government worked to decrease health spending. This time, health policymakers and planners, using sophisticated technology, were moving the health care system toward a more competitive approach to medical care based on a market model (Winn, 1987). Market demands created a whole new set of priorities that did not include community health needs. Instead, the concerns with market forces compelled providers to focus on managing health care costs and access to more expensive kinds of treatment through the rapid growth of health maintenance organizations (HMOs) and preferred provider organizations (PPOs). The impact of these new policies on poor people with historically higher rates of chronic disease and lower rates of access to regular medical care was that they were virtually excluded from obtaining access to health care, which in turn contributed to the persistence of long-standing health disparities. The result, as we know, is that government succeeded in applying the market model to Medicaid, creating the Medicaid Managed Care approach to health services for the poor, highly favored by state governments because it allows them to establish a ceiling above which Medicaid costs to the state cannot rise. Corporations also like managed care because it permits them to establish predictable budgets for employee health benefits.

At the same time that government was reducing health spending and health planners and policymakers were designing market approaches and cost containment measures for health care, a third shift in policy and resources was already under way. The 1980s saw huge increases in the cost of health technology, and many aspects of medical care became more labor-intensive. As hopeless as this situation would appear, it served as a catalyst for several of the affected groups, in urban and rural communities across the country, to begin to organize and advocate for improved health services for their communities.

Their advocacy and organizing efforts were fueled by their clarity regarding several issues. The most critical concern was that vast changes were occurring in the delivery of health services, particularly concerning availability of and access to quality care, and for the most part, these limitations were being imposed on the basis of class, which is to say, ability to pay. This meant that in the United States, where class is racialized, large numbers of poor people who are also members of ethnic and racial minority groups did not have any opportunity for input into the shape and function of these new delivery systems (Sampson, 1984).

In addition, poor people and people from nonmainstream cultures saw the managed care, HMO, and PPO systems as ineffective in meeting their needs because people in their communities were largely uninsured, did not trust Western medicine, and did not believe that the system would consider, take note of, or value their evaluations or their monitoring of the effectiveness of these new systems in their communities (Schlesinger, 1987). Finally, health advocates among the poor and the working class only had to look around them by the early 1980s to be reminded of the disinvestments in their communities and to know with certainty that the unfolding health care reforms would also be of no benefit for their communities. The result was that some communities successfully organized, negotiated for, and obtained funding to establish CBHOs and provide health services to the neediest members of their communities.

Enduring Effects of the Reagan Years

Admittedly, health care inequities did not begin with the Reagan administration. In fact, although the Nixon administration initially continued some of the work started during the War on Poverty of the Johnson years, those efforts were slowly abandoned. The one-term Carter administration was unable to interrupt the long-term disinvestment in urban areas that had technically started after World War II. As a result, inner-city residents and poor communities all across the United States continued to pay the price of government abandonment of their communities by imploding under the weight of nonfunctioning educational systems, high unemployment, escalating substance abuse, youth violence, and a disproportionate share of health and mental health problems.

As these difficulties played out in both rural and urban poor communities, they were further exacerbated by the unbalanced political and economic thrust of the Reagan years toward political and military world domination and expanding economic globalization. This focus moved the U.S. manufacturing base to cheaper suburban or overseas labor pools and diverted urban resources toward development of suburban areas and military might at the expense of services to poor people. These policies would be reinforced in later administrations irrespective of political party affiliation. This conversion in the United States from a manufacturing economy to a high-tech information and service economy, though essentially complete by 1970, was being felt deeply and dramatically in the 1980s in low-income communities. It is in these neighborhoods that the poor and low-skilled were now left without the availability of jobs in the manufacturing sector, which had customarily provided not only decent wages but also health insurance and therefore access to health care services.

The policy shifts supported by the Reagan administration represent a watershed. By the mid-1980s, Reagan's policies had become crystal-clear. They rested on a "blame the victim" approach in which the poor were expected to take responsibility for their own health, to "just say no" to any negative health behaviors, and to expect very little assistance from government. The nineteenth- and early-twentieth-century creators of public health efforts in the United States would have found this emphasis on individualism shocking, as they clearly understood that the health of a community was the key measure of its success and that if one small group or segment in the community faced disease and early death, that was a very good indication of the larger community's political and social failure (Garrett, 2000).

Lack of Access to Health Care: The Case of Immigrant Health

Immigrants provide a clear example of failures on the part of the larger society to take care of the health of a small group or segment in the community. During the early 1900s, fears about the spread of infectious diseases had abated, and by midcentury there was ample evidence that most of them had been conquered. Unfortunately, this false sense of security accounts in some ways for the situation in recent years with respect to tuberculosis (TB). The incidence of TB in the United States had been in consistent decline from 1953 until a resurgence began in 1978, due primarily to the influx of refugees from Southeast Asia as part of resettlement programs that started in the mid-1970s. Because TB screening regulations at the time had been relaxed, refugees did not undergo screening or treatment for tuberculosis before they left refugee camps (Geiter, 2000). TB is finally being brought under control again, and the most effective current methods are case management approaches that employ comprehensive, community-based, patient-centered, directly observed therapy, which achieves high treatment completion rates for TB patients (Chaulk and Kazandjian, 2003).

Despite the resurgence of this infectious disease and the need to provide immigrants with health care services, the United States has not removed the political and legal screening mechanisms imbedded in the 1965 Immigration Act that serve to bar immigrants from public benefits such as health care services. Instead, economic barriers have been added to those political and legal barriers, and, of course, the customary cultural barriers also persist. Together, these barriers serve to deny access to care. However, the more important consequence of these barriers as far as immigrants are concerned is that they have the potential to jeopardize the legal status of immigrants in the United States through punitive sanctions that can be applied not only to the immigrants but also to their sponsors.

Political and Legal Barriers

The most critical barrier is the political and legal restrictions written into the 1965 immigration legislation around the use of services. The restrictions cautioned family sponsors and their newly arrived family members of sanctions against their use of any public benefits such as Medicaid or Medicare during the first five years in the country. Not only would immigrants and their sponsors have to pay back any public monies spent on health care provided to the newcomers, but the new immigrants would also be prohibited from bringing other family members into the country, which dashes the dream of family reunification.

Economic Barriers

The economic barrier—the prohibitive cost of even basic health care—primarily affects members of the working poor, among whom are people from all groups, including a disproportionately large number of immigrants and other people of color. By the 1970s, the cost of health care delivery was skyrocketing out of control. The initial response, starting with the Nixon administration in the early 1970s, was to institute economic controls to bring down health care costs for employers: HMO legislation was enacted along with coinsurance, which allows employers to share health care costs with employees; deductibles, which establish thresholds below which employer-sponsored health insurance is not responsible for covering costs; and other measures aimed at halting runaway health costs for employers.

These economic controls had a dire effect on all members of the working poor. For example, even when the working poor have jobs that provide health insurance, the costs of deductibles, coinsurance, prescription medications, and other out-of-pocket expenses associated with long-term chronic disease are not always affordable. And the situation is worse for members of the working poor who are not in jobs that provide health benefits. The cost of health insurance is prohibitive, and they do not make enough money to purchase health insurance on their own.

Cultural Barriers

Cultural barriers, unlike political and legal or economic screens, have a more profound and far-reaching negative impact on all racial and ethnically different people living in the United States. The Hart-Cellar Immigration Act of 1965 was a major turning point in that it represented the first time in U.S. history that immigration policy allowed the entry of large numbers of people who were not only racially and ethnically different from the mainstream but also culturally different. At the same time, the more critical issue here, given U.S. history, is that the new policies, allowing the entry of newcomers with racial, ethnic, linguistic, and cultural differences, were not accompanied by a new mind-set or any sort of widespread effort to manage differences or to change Americans' perceptions. Outdated attitudes persist, whereby newcomers are viewed not in terms of the rich diversity they bring and the many resources they contribute to the nation but rather in terms of their difference from the mainstream.

Also outdated but equally persistent are the harmful divisions that marginalized groups erect among themselves, as is the case with people of African ancestry in the United States. At a recent meeting in Maryland to develop plans for the education of African Americans about the dangers of prostate cancer, an Ethiopian-born black man was told that the education efforts would focus only on native-born blacks, not on any others. The debate over heritage or who has a legitimate claim to the term *African American* in this instance is irrelevant when the issues being considered are the dangers of prostate cancer, the need for communitywide education, health care for all, or even more urgently, life and death (Swarns, 2004).

Early in U.S. history, in addition to the forced immigration of slaves, American immigration policy was one of open borders as the colonies and later the nation welcomed all who could help build it. As immigration levels increased during the second half of the nineteenth century, so did xenophobia—hostility toward foreigners or outsiders—which became focused on Chinese immigrants. This led to the Chinese Exclusion Act of 1882, followed by a ten-year ban on immigration from China. U.S. immigration policy has essentially remained very conservative with the exception of the period initiated by the 1965 Immigration Act. Since then, immigration reforms that began in 1985 have been largely built on conservative policies opposing immigration. These policies have now become even more stringent since the tragic events of September 11, 2001.

The conservatism in immigration policy was motivated by racism, and U.S. policy long gave preferences to immigrants from European countries, allowing entry by only small numbers of nonwhites each year. The rationale for the preferential treatment of Europeans was "assimilability," the assumed easier integration of persons from countries with historical, racial, cultural, and linguistic traditions similar to those already here (New York City Department of City Planning, 1996). The result of that kind of thinking, as we have seen, was the development of the barriers enacted in 1965 and reinforced throughout the past four decades.

The conservative thinking that has guided immigration policy continues to limit the ability of all people in the United States who are poor, are racially or ethnically different, be they native-born or immigrant, or are uninsured to obtain the health services required to maintain or improve their health. These barriers also make it evident that the traditional medical model of health care delivery would not be effective in providing services for groups that are not part of the U.S. mainstream.

The Impact of Policy Changes on CBHOs

Before there were political and economic indications of the need for CBHOs, there was evidence that there had been a shift in the types of diseases we were confronting, especially among the mainstream population. This shift was first solidified early in the twentieth century after conducting health screening of U.S. soldiers in preparation for World War I. Those screenings yielded data substantiating that the United States had begun to experience a higher incidence of chronic diseases, which was quite a change from the acute and sudden infectious episodes of the recent past. Despite variations in the extent to which chronic disease can be prevented or treated, two proven activities are important to the prevention and early detection and treatment of chronic diseases: public health education and screening for multiple illnesses by local health entities (Warren, 1965).

Health education was one of the early casualties of health care cutbacks in the 1980s and 1990s. During that time, health care advocates, minority health professionals, and advocates for poor and minority communities knew that the health problems in poor communities could not be separated from the lack of information in those communities about prevention practices, in addition to the many other burdens borne by those communities. Poverty and high unemployment have long been associated with high levels of drug abuse, violent crime, teen pregnancies, and poor health (McBarnette, 1996). Poverty in particular is closely associated with an excess of preventable deaths that begin in infancy and extend throughout the life cycle (Bayne Smith and Perot, 2003).

The decision by community residents to establish a CBHO is almost always made in response to a crisis. Indeed, in previous centuries, it was the crisis conditions of communicable diseases that precipitated the establishment of a permanent board of health in New York City. As a result, when faced with reduced spending on health care and other resources for the poor, the lack of health education and information in their communities, and the absence of regular sources of ongoing, culturally appropriate health care, several communities took steps to protect their own health by developing their own CBHOs.

The establishment of CBHOs, like any service offered in cities, is almost always related to the financial situation of the city in which that CBHO is located, and as we know, cities are themselves affected by what is happening at the state and national levels. However, economic conditions, whether in times of comfort or of crisis, are essentially political events that are driven by interest group conflicts and negotiations about not only how best to divide the pie but also how to pay for it. The health care pie is no exception. In fact, health care services, from the smallest CBHO to the large medical center, are politically and economically contested entities as health care embodies the intersection of public and private sectors of the economy. Large health care organizations such as hospitals rely equally on government support in the form of payments from Medicare, Medicaid, and the Child Health Insurance Program and private support from commercial insurance, out-of-pocket payments, or private philanthropy and foundations that fund special health projects and programs.

As a result of the intense political and economic interest that CBHOs generate, they tend to be established not as independent entities in any given city but as part of the general political and economic structure of the city. CBHOs that are federally funded 330 facilities and that provide clinical services bring federal monies into their community and thereby contribute to the financial condition of their city. Those, along with other kinds of CBHOs, are often at the center of hotly debated political negotiations and attempts at collaborations as the federal dollars they bring are coveted by a host of other health care agencies. Some cities and states, exercising creative management, have been able to foster cooperative use of federal 330 money by establishing so-called primary care development corporations (PCDCs). The charge to PCDCs is to maximize the use of federal dollars by negotiating partnerships and collaborations between community groups who have been awarded 330 funding and state, municipal, or voluntary hospitals, with the goal of providing access or outright control of those dollars not to the CBHO but in reality to the hospital entity, irrespective of whether it is a state, municipal, or voluntary institution.

Transferring Health Services from Government to the Nonprofit Sector

Just as the federal government began in earnest in the 1980s to transfer responsibility for resident services to the states and cities, cities have likewise passed the responsibility for resident services on to nonprofits. According to the Center for Technology in Government (2003), local governments began to transfer nonessential functions to private companies by the late 1980s. By the 1990s, states routinely privatized traditional types of governmental functions, such as the construction and operation of prison systems. This has met with mixed reactions, as private owners of prisons are able to use prison labor for profitmaking. The more widely accepted current form of government transfer of responsibility for services has been in the human services arena. In this case, government establishes a contractual agreement with nonprofit service agencies to deliver a preagreed package of services, within a specific time frame, to eligible recipients.

This transfer of social and health services from government to nonprofits has succeeded primarily for two reasons. First, devolution has been interpreted as a unique business opportunity, especially by larger nonprofits with the resources to develop programs and lobby government to eventually institutionalize those programs or at the very least to commit to providing support as long as it was politically feasible to do so. Second, giving from the private sector, especially from private philanthropy, and corporate giving steadily increased from the 1970s into the new century. The recent dip in corporate and foundation grants to the nonprofit world has been attributed to the combined effects of the terrorist attacks of September 11, 2001, and the subsequent economic downturn.

The oldest examples of a responsibility transfer arrangement are to be found in the GI Bill. After World War II, U.S. soldiers obtained educational benefits that entitled them to go to college under the GI Bill, which paid a portion of their tuition and fees for attending an accredited institution of higher learning. Research indicates that even before the New Deal, grants were being used at the federal level to transfer resources to the states, and these grants have always been tied to the political climate at any given moment in history (Salamon, 1989). However, over the past forty years, states have imitated federal behavior by steadily increasing government contracts to nonprofits to provide social services. However, whenever governments cut back the amount of funding they provide to nonprofits, they create a crisis in the nonprofits' ability to meet service demands in the community (Salamon, 1996).

Government contracting with nonprofits throughout the years has of course included CBHOs, and with good reason. There are multiple advantages to working with CBHOs, as they are capable of penetrating their communities at much deeper levels than outsiders and can develop culturally and linguistically appropriate health promotion messages that will resonate in their communities (Remine, Rice, and Ross, 1984; Delgado, 2002). CBHOs enter into contractual agreements with government because providing health and health-related services to their community is in keeping with their organizational mission and vision and also because in obtaining contracts and grants, CBHOs provide employment, thereby contributing to the economic development of their communities. At first glance, this appears to be an ideal public-community partnership. Closer examination reveals that the survival of CBHOs is constantly under attack due largely to the economic and political aspects of their relationship to government entities.

CBHO-Government Relations: The Impact of Economic and Political Policies

It is becoming increasingly clear that CBHOs must continue to play a vital role as partners in the public health arena and that they have done effective work in specific areas such as helping control the spread of sexually transmitted disease (Klein, Birkhead, and Murphy, 1998), increasing community immunization rates, (Irigoyen and Findley, 1998), and making effective use of community health workers who can educate their community as well as health providers (Horowitz, Davis, Palermo, and Vladeck, 2000).

Despite their successes to date, CBHOs remain heavily dependent on government grants, which do not provide resources or training for organizational capacity building in critical areas such as improved technological capability and training, data collection, or documentation. The impact of these inadequate aspects of government funding is that it renders CBHOs incapable of assessing their contributions to improved health outcomes (Irigoyen and Findley, 1998) and creates the impression of unintentionally (some would say intentionally) destabilizing CBHOs. Whatever the intent, the terms and conditions of government funding make it difficult for CBHOs to argue their worth or make any demands on government. In a high-tech, data-driven society, this places CBHOs at risk of losing funding and ultimately threatens the very survival of their agencies.

A major area of strain in the relationship between CBHOs and government has to do with the cumbersome procedures that large government bureaucracies employ in their reimbursement systems. States exercise full control over monies received from the federal government for programs in terms of the actual amounts of money distributed to local agencies as well as the timeliness of those distributions. As a result, a CBHO may successfully compete for a grant through the request for proposals or request for applications process, receive notification that it has been awarded a grant, and yet not receive a penny of that grant for six or more months.

Yet some states require that program implementation begin at the time of notification of the grant award, even though no monies to implement the grant have been disbursed by the state. Program implementation necessitates financial expenditures that small, grant-dependent CBHOs are not always capable of providing. One solution some CBHOs have employed is to obtain a line of credit from their local bank. However, budgets of most government grants do not include a line item for interest payment on loans. Some CBHOs are able to develop strategies for managing these financial burdens, but others buckle under the weight of constant financial strains.

Another threat to continued CBHO existence in a Medicaid Managed Care (MMC) environment is that while some states demand that every indigent person join a managed care program in order to obtain care, these states do not require that the MMC companies partner with the CBHOs that have been serving as the trusted providers of care in their community prior to the arrival of MMC. Moreover, CBHOs continue to struggle with delivering services to constituents who have been affected by federal social reforms, specifically welfare reform and immigration reform.

Welfare Reform

In 1935, the United States established a welfare system known as Aid to Families with Dependent Children (AFDC). This harsh and punitive program was eventually eliminated when President Clinton signed the Personal Responsibility and Work Opportunity Reconciliation Act (PRWORA) into law in August 1996. In October 1996, a new federal program, Temporary Assistance for Needy Families (TANF), replaced AFDC. The intent of PRWORA was to provide training for women coming off AFDC to prepare them to enter the labor market, and TANF would provide short-term assistance in the event that parents could not find work to tide them over until they resumed employment. The problem, however, is that in some states, welfare reform had already begun prior to the implementation of these two laws, and those states were making significant strides in enforcing policies designed to encourage both old and new applicants to seek work and leave the welfare rolls.

Support for the new direction taken by various states was provided by PRWORA and TANF as these two pieces of legislation caused three major changes in the lives of poor women and children. First, states were required to reduce their number of welfare recipients by 50 percent by 2002 by involving them in some work-related program or activity. Second, TANF put in place specific time limits for receiving cash income from the government. Third, these policies separated enrollment of recipients in welfare and in Medicaid.

Efforts to decrease the rolls were quite successful, with all states meeting the federal welfare-to-work requirements by 1998. The larger problem for most states has been keeping poor women in work-related situations. TANF imposed a five-year lifetime limit on receiving federal assistance, but research has shown that people have high rates of recidivism, going on and off welfare for a variety of reasons that include low levels of education, inadequate job skills, and lack of adequate child care or paid sick leave that would enable them to stay home and take care of a sick child (Kneipp, 2000).

The more immediate problem for former welfare recipients in terms of access to health care is to be found in the separation of TANF from Medicaid eligibility. As people exited the welfare caseloads, some states, using cost-saving devices, were not forthcoming in notifying many women that they and their children would still qualify for Medicaid or at the very least their children would qualify for the federal Child Health Insurance Program. By not informing former welfare recipients of their eligibility for Medicaid and connecting them to a medical home that in some cases would have to be an MMC organization, those states in essence erected significant barriers to access to preventive health care and in some cases to urgently needed acute care for indigent families.

The impact of welfare reform on the mission statements and values of many CBHOs forced them to develop another set of skills in the advocacy arena. CBHOs have begun to collaborate with social justice organizations and some national foundations to put pressure on elected officials in the more recalcitrant states to account for and more effectively use Medicaid block grant dollars to increase local outreach, education, and enrollment in Medicaid and CHIP. Data from the Kaiser Foundation Commission on Medicaid provide a state-by-state breakout indicating that these efforts have succeeded in increasing Medicaid and CHIP enrollment. The Kaiser state-level information can be found at http://www.kff.org.

Immigration Reform

The harsh barriers to health care access embedded in the 1965 Hart-Cellar Act pales in comparison to the more stringent restrictions later imposed by the combined political and legal force of immigration and welfare reforms of the 1990s. The Personal Responsibility and Work Reconciliation Act of 1996, commonly referred to as welfare reform, divides immigrants into "qualified" and "unqualified" aliens. "Qualified" aliens include primarily immigrants who are legal permanent residents or green card holders, refugees, and asylees. However, there are further distinctions. A qualified immigrant who had entered the United States before August 22, 1996, would be eligible for Medicaid coverage for health care services and for the newly reconfigured TANF program only after residing in the country for five years.

If an immigrant participated in a public assistance program, his or her sponsor becomes responsible for the reimbursement of any public dollars spent on health care for the immigrant. Individuals in this same group of qualified immigrants would also be eligible for other public benefits, including food stamps, state food assistance, and Supplemental Security Income if they met other criteria (child under age eighteen legally in the United States, refugee, disabled). On the contrary, qualified immigrants arriving in the United States after August 1996 were eligible for TANF, Medicaid, food stamps, and other benefits only if the immigrant fit into a specific immigration classification (refugee, asylee, person granted withholding of deportation, veteran of active military duty or family member of such, member of certain categories of Native Americans) and did not use any of these public benefits outside of defined time periods. Needless to say, the restrictions on "unqualified" aliens were more severely designed so as to render them ineligible for anything but emergency Medicaid.

One glaring example of how immigration reform places the burden of health disparities on the shoulders of immigrants and the poor is provided by the infant mortality rate (IMR) in New York City. As noted in earlier chapters, the IMR is the number of infant deaths per thousand live births. In 1999, the IMR in New York was at a record low of 6.8. However, the IMR in communities around the city with heavy concentrations of immigrant populations was as high as 12, compared to IMRs as low as 1.9 in city neighborhoods that are predominantly white and middle-class. Furthermore, when the IMR data were analyzed in greater detail, the results indicated that the top five groups with the highest IMRs were all of African ancestry, both native and foreign-born (Katz, 1999).

Welfare and immigration reform diminished the ability of CBHOs to provide services to the various subpopulations they customarily serve in several ways, from denying access to care for the neediest to short-circuiting health care spending. Together, these policy reforms sent a very loud message: government wants to provide less costly services to fewer people with the expectation that the nonprofit sector will pick up the slack (Abramson and Salamon, 1986). By denying Medicaid coverage to poor women exiting the welfare rolls and to immigrants, the United States effectively denied coverage to ongoing preventive health care, which leads to several other problems. First, lack of health coverage and access to care supports negative health practices that contribute to health disparities. When access to care through Medicaid is denied, the tendency among the poor is to wait until their health situation is unbearable and then obtain care in emergency rooms, at which point they qualify for emergency Medicaid. Second, the expensive cost of using the emergency room and its acute-care medical model to provide care for chronic diseases contributes in large measure both to the high cost of health care expenditures and to the persistence of health disparities.

Political Strategies for CBHOs

The survival of CBHOs in the kind of political and economic climate described in this chapter calls for different political strategies that at least hold out hope that CBHOs will be able to continue to serve their communities. Now much more than they ever did before, CBHOs need new political approaches in handling the difficult issues surrounding the responsibility for service delivery based on government grants and contracts as well as the perilous nature of grant dependency. The need for CBHOs to reassess and if need be renegotiate their relationship with funding sources is directly related to critical changes in social spending that have been implemented by the administration of President George W. Bush. Although the Bush administration did not initiate cuts in Medicaid spending, it added to the policy conflict by restructuring Medicaid.

The Bush administration seized on the year-old Medicare-based ceiling known as the "upper payment limit" (UPL) that the Clinton administration had imposed in October 2000 to reduce Medicaid payments to the states to 150 percent of comparable Medicare payments to hospitals, nursing facilities, clinics, and intermediate care facilities for the mentally ill. In January 2001, the Bush administration reduced the UPL to 100 percent and gave the states two years, until March 19, 2003, to come into compliance with the new ruling. Although the various professional associations representing hospitals sought an injunction to stop the Bush administration's implementation date, a judge eventually ruled that the lowered UPL established by the Bush administration would go into effect immediately (Matherlee, 2002).

Undeniably, the states were using loopholes under the Clinton era UPL to drive up the federal Medicaid matching funds they received. However, the solution need not have been to lower the UPL further. Instead, it would have been more beneficial to the health of poor people if the Bush administration had instituted uniform accounting measures that would prevent creative efforts by the states to increase their share of federal revenue, sanctions against states that accessed more Medicaid dollars than they were entitled to, and stringent measures to ensure that the federal Medicaid dollars the states did obtain were used solely to provide appropriate services for their indigent residents.

The implication for CBHOs and the clients they serve of lowered federal Medicaid payments to the states is essentially that less money is available overall to provide health care for the indigent. This then translates into reduced funding for programs and services to community residents, as there will ultimately be reductions not only in the numbers of state contracts awarded but also in the dollar amount of each contract. Indeed, all health and health-related providers, including physicians and hospitals, are also likely to be hit with reduced funding. However, CBHOs, especially those that are not 330 clinics and are serving the poor, immigrants, racial and ethnic minorities, and the disempowered, are at an even greater disadvantage. They simply cannot begin to match the level of organization and capacity to lobby and otherwise bring pressure to bear on policymakers that hospitals, doctors, and even some clinics can.

Political Realities for CBHOs

Most CBHOs, particularly if they receive government funding, do not operate outside of the political environment. In fact, the political strategy of most CBHOs that obtain government funding is built around their ability to effectively communicate to elected officials the importance of awarding contracts to provide services for a community of voters. It is not realistic to expect to obtain funding, in a health care environment of diminished resources, without at the very least developing some level of relationship with the decision makers who determine how resources are to be distributed.

Structurally, most CBHOs are nonprofits. As such, they are legally allowed to conduct voter registration drives, as that is nonpartisan activity. It is crucially important for CBHOs to clearly understand that there are legal sanctions against them if they engage in political activity to support specific candidates. The problem they face is that in resource-strapped cities, the powerful business sector will obtain concessions from government, as will other interest groups, and if CBHOs do not have a political strategy to ensure that their voices are heard, they will not be able to meet the needs of their community. Therefore, CBHOs, like all others who seek support from government, must do more than simply make their voices heard.

An important step for CBHOs is to first understand the ways in which government decision making about the distribution of resources helps foster competition for resources among various groups. Next, CBHOs are being called on more and more to organize their communities and develop strong advocates among the clients they serve. Finally, they must also strategically position themselves within policymaking circles so that pressure on political decision making regarding resource distribution can be exerted from both within as well as outside the system.

The Zero-Sum Game

Political decision making about who gets what from government, in the larger sense, is about issues of power and control: control over what decisions are made and who makes them, what resources are distributed, how much is given, to whom, and for what purposes. In the same way that business leaders, community groups, and others attempt to control the outcomes of decisions, the decision makers themselves are concerned with exercising control as well. Decision makers are more likely to seize control over decisions that affect poor people or those who are perceived as having little or no power, and they do so by engaging in various methods of psychological manipulation. One such method is known as the zero-sum game.

According to the zero-sum belief, any gains provided to one group or individual come at the expense of another group or individual. In other words, in a world of limited resources, providing any resources to one group is possible only by taking resources away from another group. When CBHOs or any community group accepts the zero-sum model, several negative outcomes result. In extreme cases, the CBHO and its community in effect give up their goals of improved health, individual and community empowerment, and community economic development, leaving full power and control over resources in the hands of the decision makers. In other situations, the CBHO and its community may focus on fighting more powerful business groups or, worse, fighting other CBHOs and poor communities for a few small crumbs.

The antidote to zero-sum thinking is to recognize it for what it is: psychological manipulation to control valuable community energy and resources by directing them against a "competitor." The more rational approach is to expand the request. Incorporate the needs of the other CBHOs into one request, thereby turning the zero-sum game into a win-win situation for community groups and an opportunity for collaboration. In this way, groups that were being pitted against each other can collectively pressure those in power to meet the needs of the communities they were elected to serve. This is a much more progressive approach. To operate in this manner, however, CBHOs have to be cognizant that three critical factors—the circumstances of an issue, the locus of power, and control of that particular issue—are constantly changing. All three factors are very much dependent on the situation in question, and the solution must be non-zero-sum.

Effective Political Strategies

One advantageous political strategy for many CBHOs that does not violate the requirements of their nonprofit status is to broadly conduct voter registration drives as a vehicle for organizing and mobilizing their community. However, they must encourage voter participation in the electoral process in a nonpartisan manner.

At the same time, individuals in leadership positions, board members, and organized committees that are "friends of" the CBHO may privately, as U.S. citizens, engage in voter organization, delivering a "constituency," if possible, to one or two carefully selected candidates who have been helpful or have the potential to be helpful to the CBHO by virtue of the kinds of policymaking committees on which they sit in the state legislature, city council, or Congress. In addition, individual friends or board members may also serve specific candidates and elected officials in an advisory capacity. In this fashion, the CBHO enhances its ability to influence decision making regarding grants and contracts from within. At the same time, voter registration allows CBHOs to organize and mobilize the community so that if need be, pressure can also be brought to bear from without.

Although some CBHOs have worked openly to organize voters on behalf of a particular candidate, this is not advisable, even though these organizations may for a time enjoy tremendous influence over decision making. Remember that issues of political control, decision making, and power are always changing.

An even more valuable tool in the CBHO arsenal of political strategies involves building and maintaining relationships to the community being served, building relationships with the elected officials who represent that community, and most important, building relationships between these two entities. For example, CBHOs can benefit from institutionalizing a once- or twice-a-year "community and legislative breakfast meeting" or similar event in which the CBHO provides the forum for the community to come together with elected officials and government agency representatives. This can be a well-organized opportunity for decision makers to see the strength in numbers and hear directly from the CBHOs' constituency. It is also the kind of event at which all elected representatives will want to put in an appearance so as to make use of a photo opportunity and press coverage and where with careful organization, the community can extract a commitment from the decision makers not only for continued funding for needed services but also to work with the community toward empowerment, economic development, and long-term self sufficiency.

This political strategy of bringing together community members and the decision makers elected to represent them is particularly important because the most critical challenge for CBHOs is their ability to build and sustain credible internal capacity for influencing the debate at the policy table (Markham, 1998). The work of bringing the electorate closer to the elected is now part and parcel of the advocacy function of CBHOs. CBHOs who are able to influence the debate at the policy level possess two critical characteristics. They have earned the trust of the people they serve, and they have also earned the kind of respect from others in the larger sociopolitical environment that only comes from being viewed as credible and reliable. When CBHOs possess these two traits, they have the currency that buys them a seat at the policy table and places them in the position of being sought out for policy input.

In discussing some of the helpful political strategies that CBHOs can use to more effectively obtain funding to serve their communities, it is evident that implementation of these strategies involves time, skills, and abilities that are separate from service delivery, program development, and management and from the mission and commitment to serve a community. Political strategies are much more connected on the one hand to ensuring and building community capacity to negotiate from an empowered position. On the other hand, political strategies are now vital to building organizational capacity to deliver services. The difficulty for most CBHOs is striking a balance between these two very different sets of skills and activities.

Achieving Balance: Commitment to Serve Versus Capacity to Serve

In connection with the research reported on in Chapter Three, several in-depth interviews with staff members at CBHOs were conducted. The interviews provided rich information, most often about the commitment of the individuals initially involved in the usual struggles that accompany the establishment of CBHOs. In almost every case, what came through was the willingness of a single individual to bring these large projects to fruition, often with nothing more than a desire to serve a particular population or group. Although the level of commitment our interviewees described is certainly laudable, it is important to recognize that commitment and passion alone are not enough.

Administrators interviewed at growing and successful CBHOs that had been in existence for twenty or more years also made it quite clear that along with the commitment to serve, they either brought with them or were forced to quickly develop another level of expertise. All of these administrators repeatedly pointed out that there have been critical changes in terms of the set of skills and personal resources that are now required for managing a CBHO. It is now necessary to not only build but also sustain sufficient organizational capacity if programs and indeed entire organizations are to survive. And regrettably, funding for building organizational capacity, from public or private sources, is almost nonexistent.

Staying True to the Mission

Some of the earliest work that any CBHO engages in is the development of its mission and vision and the determination of its core values. This is the groundwork, the essentials, the fundamental basis on which the organization rests, and all else flows from this early work. However, all living organisms are constantly evolving, and organizations are no exception. The challenge for CBHOs as they grow and evolve is to be mindful of staying true to their mission or else changing it to reflect new realities. If the mission is to truly guide the course of the organization, it will also guide decisions about what kinds of funding to pursue and from whom. This becomes particularly difficult as organizations that are struggling to survive may find themselves having to refuse specific kinds of funding that would conflict with their organizational mission.

For example, should an organization that provides maternal child health services accept funding from a tobacco company or from a company that sells alcoholic beverages? How would doing so affect the credibility of the organization? Should a CBHO that provides HIV/AIDS services to a broad cross section of infected and affected adults and children accept a large donation from a recording artist who is an avowed homophobe? Staying true to the mission is larger than simply doing what is politically correct in programming or staffing. It is much more important to be coherent and consistent in terms of mission, vision, values, programs, and funding.

Steering the Organizational Course

The leaders of CBHOs engage in daily political and economic struggles in a health care environment that is best described as hostile. Externally, they face inordinate amounts of pressure from government funding sources to provide more services on less money. In the external environment, CBHOs are increasingly competing with corporations that have now entered the nonprofit service market, bringing with them the type of business management acumen that small CBHOs simply do not have. Finally, the lack of technological skills in data collection and performance measurement discussed earlier is a critical drawback in competing for clients, funding, and other resources in today's health care arena.

Needless to say, CBHOs cannot survive without building strong internal organizational capacity, which is vital to the management of programs, funding, marketing of the organization, and long-term sustainability. These requirements for internal development are discussed in Chapter Six; however, the impact of the political and economic constraints discussed in this chapter on the commitment and capacity of CBHOs to serve their communities requires a focused response in two major areas that may be new to many CBHOs: the development of an advocacy function and building of cross-organizational collaborations, even at times with competing organizations.

The Advocacy Function of CBHOs

There are currently no indications that the impact of policy changes on CBHOs and the diminished funding levels that have resulted are likely to improve in the near future. This situation makes it imperative that CBHOs develop new strategies, skills, and functions for obtaining required resources to meet the health needs of their communities. One of the many roles or functions that managers of CBOs and CBHOs have now undertaken is that of advocacy. As noted in Chapter One, an advocate is an individual who works for people with problems, and these are often people who are extremely difficult to organize (Rubin and Rubin, 1992).

Advocacy involves outreach and recruitment to bring people together, preferably as members of organizations, to stage protest demonstrations, make telephone calls, write letters, send fax blitzes, or otherwise lobby a policymaker on behalf of their group or organization, all toward goals such as policy change or increased resources to address identified needs. During the early days of organizing in labor unions and the civil rights movement, for example, advocacy was frequently used by groups seeking change, whether nationally or at the neighborhood level.

Although advocacy continues to employ some of the earlier activities, it now includes very sophisticated strategies that run the gamut from communitywide accountability meetings with elected officials to legal action against government to secure benefits for citizens. The emphasis is clearly on influencing the political system to function in ways that benefit the entire citizenry, because long-term positive benefits for poor people are unlikely to occur without concerted efforts aimed not only at policy change but also the subsequent implementation of policy in helpful rather than harmful ways.

As a result, advocacy is now a crucial function for CBHOs, particularly those that are grant-dependent, because it provides a more promising and more confident approach for providing policymakers with information from the communities they are elected to serve and for pressuring decision makers to increase health care funding. Advocacy can also serve the larger organizational need to use media effectively for the purposes of shaping public opinion and political agendas while also maintaining a high profile, which helps to keep the organization in the news and in the minds and hearts of clients, competitors, policymakers, and other funding sources.

Developing an advocacy function can be onerous, particularly for the administrators of CBHOs with whom responsibility for development of advocacy strategies will ultimately rest. CBHOs advocacy strategies will have to include constituency outreach, education, recruitment, and organizing, as well as training and building leadership among constituents, whose collective voices have the potential to be far more powerful than any administrator who would speak on their behalf. Some CBHOs have been able to incorporate advocacy into the very fabric of their organizational mission and efforts. For example, a CBHO in Rhode Island has developed a constituent member organization of some eight hundred dues-paying individuals and families in their neighborhood (the dues are nominal—$5 per individual or per family per year) . In another case, outreach, engagement, and education of the clients they serve is a fundamental aspect of the advocacy efforts of La Clinica del Pueblo in Washington, D.C., whose director believes that consumers and community residents are the best advocates the clinic could have (Bayne Smith and Perot, 2003).

Given the time and skills required to successfully develop and implement an advocacy function, two recommendations are worthy of consideration here. First, advocacy ought not to be the bailiwick of only the managerial staff. It should become a function of the board of directors, with a board-level committee that works with managers to develop plans and strategies for advocacy. Second, as a protective measure, single CBHOs, especially the smaller ones, should not go it alone. Advocacy is always more successful on the sheer strength of numbers. Therefore, plans and strategies to accomplish this function will benefit from careful decisions about collaboration and building coalitions for advocacy, even with competitors.

Building Collaborations

CBHOs, especially in their initial stages, tend to be the product of an individual or a small group of people who work extremely hard to bring a vision to fruition. Indeed, part of the success of small neighborhood-based CBHOs comes from the fact that thanks to their size, they are able to focus on neighborhood projects and accomplish them in clear and visible ways that garner community support. However, when CBHOs need to tackle formidable, structural issues affecting their community that are economically and politically based, they benefit more from the collective muscle, skills, data, and technological capabilities that other (sometimes statewide or national) organizations can bring to a collaborative effort. Currently, CBHOs and other nonprofits all face similar difficulties in terms of diminishing funding. Collaborations provide a much less costly means of providing such benefits to staff as health insurance and training and a much more cost-effective method of providing and expanding services, collecting and analyzing data, and planning and carrying out more powerful advocacy strategies.

Although there are multiple advantages to collaboration when distinct organizations decide to work together, careful decisions have to be made about the nature of such relationships that will depend on the magnitude of the problem to be addressed, the distinctive characteristics of the groups to be included, and the type and amount of resources required. This kind of information will assist in development of the most effective governance format to achieve the goals of the collaboration. A variety of models exists for building collaborations. For issues on which short-term cooperation is needed, a less formal model is needed. When organizations plan to work together over the long haul, there is a need for clarity before signing a formal agreement and committing to becoming a member of a team, whether it be a network, an alliance, or a coalition. Assurances of long-term compatibility ought to flow from a thorough check of each organization's willingness to share information, ideas, and skills and an even more thorough assessment of how closely they are aligned on goals as well as the level of tolerance they have for differences in tactics and methods and resource commitments, including money.

Probably the greatest caution to be exercised in developing collaborations is to ensure and protect each organization from being co-opted by larger, stronger organizations and in the process becoming dependent and losing their unique identity. Nevertheless, the benefits of collaboration are critical to the survival of CBHOs, and so as they enter into collaborative arrangements, they need do so in a protective manner. CBHOs will have to find issues of common interest while not losing sight of their commitment to serve their community and the pursuit of their organizational goals.

Conclusion

The political and economic environment of CBHOs has been particularly perilous, fraught with harsh policies, increased demands, heightened competition, and dwindling resources. Some of these policies, instituted initially at the federal level and copied at the local level, have been especially injurious to CBHOs because even as they are operating with diminished resources as part of "devolution," the demand for services continues to increase. As a survival mechanism, some CBHOs have been able to develop highly evolved skill sets that they use to organize and build their communities to become involved in advocating for needed resources. They have also had to develop collaborations, sometimes with competing organizations, to capitalize on their joint resources and energies to pressure policymakers and decision makers into providing more resources to meet community health needs.

Consequently, the advocacy function of CBHOs is now an integral part of the skills that they bring to bear on community health and on the sustainability of their institutions and by extension the sustainability of the communities in which they operate.

Key Points

- CBHOs are positively or adversely affected by their political and economic environment, depending on their level of skill in navigating that environment.
- Conservative fiscal and social (immigration) policies instituted in the past forty years continue to restrict health care access in communities inhabited by the poor, racial and ethnic minorities, and immigrants.
- In the first phase of devolution, the federal government transferred to the states responsibilities for providing social services to citizens. In the second phase, state and city governments transferred that responsibility to the nonprofit sector and provided even fewer resources. This process has resulted in weakening CBHOs structurally and programmatically.

- CBHOs must now focus not only on organizational management of programs and other services but also on political and economic advocacy if they are to secure needed resources. As they engage in advocacy, some CBHOs are organizing their constituents to assist in this effort.
- CBHOs must also develop broader coalitions and collaborations to garner the necessary political power to create changes both within and outside the community.
- The major challenge for CBHOs is to maintain a balance between their commitment to serve the community and the reality of their capacity to serve.

Study Questions

1. City budgets are a matter of public record. Compare the budgets of the city or locality you live in for the past three years to identify how much money was budgeted in each of those years for three departments or agencies: health, police, and fire. Which departments experienced an increase, a decrease, or no change in their annual budgets over the three years? Based on the discussion in this chapter, provide an analysis of why budgetary changes occurred in any of these areas.
2. Find an existing coalition of health organizations in your geographical area. Some of the most active ones tend to be in the health areas of HIV/AIDS and maternal child health. Obtain an appointment to conduct a brief (twenty-minute) interview with a member of the coalition's steering committee. In that interview, you want to obtain answers to three questions: What is the purpose of the coalition, the reason for collaborating? Who are the member agencies and organizations, what does each contribute, and how does each benefit? What advocacy strategies are being employed to strengthen the coalition and its member agencies?
3. Identify a CBHO in your city or locality that has been in existence for at least ten years. Get a copy of its annual report or any document that describes the organization. Look at its current mission statement, and carefully study the programs and services the organization offer. How true to its mission has the organization stayed? Justify your answer with examples.

References

Abramson, A. J., and Salamon, L. M. *The Nonprofit Sector and the New Federal Budget.* Washington, D.C.: Urban Institute Press, 1986.

Bayne Smith, M. A., and Perot, R. T. *Report of Environmental Scan of Consumer Advocacy Needs and Requirements in the District of Columbia.* Washington, D.C.: Consumer Health Foundation, 2003.

Center for Technology in Government. *New Models of Collaboration for Public Service Delivery: Current Status of Collaboration in Selected Countries.* Washington, D.C.: Center for Technology in Government, 2003.

Chaulk, C. P., and Kazandjian, V. A. "Comprehensive Case Management Models for Pulmonary Tuberculosis." Unpublished manuscript, 2003.

Conservation Company. *HIV Health and Human Services Planning Council of New York: Needs Assessment.* New York: Conservation Company, 2000.

Delgado, D. Y. *The Plain Talk Implementation Guide: Tools for Developing Community Programs to Reduce Teen Pregnancy, STDs, and HIV/AIDS.* Baltimore: Annie E. Casey Foundation, 2002.

Dutton, D. B. "Social Class, Health, and Illness." In L. H. Aiken and D. Mechanic (eds.), *Applications of Social Science to Clinical Medicine and Health Policy.* New Brunswick, N.J.: Rutgers University Press, 1987.

Eaton, L. "Behind a Troubled Bench: An Arcane Way of Picking Judges." *New York Times,* June 30, 2003, p. B9.

Garrett, L. *Betrayal of Trust: The Collapse of Global Public Health.* New York: Hyperion, 2000.

Geiter, L. (ed.). *Ending Neglect: The Elimination of Tuberculosis in the United States.* Washington, D.C.: National Academy Press, 2000.

Horowitz, C. R., Davis, M. H., Palermo, A. S., and Vladeck, B. C. "Approaches to Eliminating Socio-Cultural Disparities in Health." *Health Care Financing Review,* 2000, *21*(4), 57–74.

Irigoyen, M., and Findley, S. E. "Methodological Difficulties in Assessing Contributions by Community-Based Organizations to Improving Child Health." Editorial. *Archives of Pediatric and Adolescent Medicine,* 1998, *152,* 318–320.

Katz, N. L. "Fear Kills Immigrant Babies." *Daily News,* Nov. 28, 1999, p. 4.

Klein, S. J., Birkhead, G. S., and Murphy, D. P. "Role of Community-Based Organizations in Control of Sexually Transmitted Diseases." Letter to the editor. *Journal of the American Medical Association,* 1998, *280,* 419.

Kneipp, S. "The Consequences of Welfare Reform for Women's Health: Issues of Concern for Community Health Nursing." *Journal of Community Health and Nursing,* 2000, *17*(2), 65–73.

Markham, D. C. "Maintaining Our Place at the Table." *American Forests,* 1998, *103*(4), 47.

Matherlee, K. *The Federal-State Struggle over Medicaid Matching Funds: An Update.* Washington, D.C.: National Health Policy Forum, 2002.

McBarnette, L. S. "African American Women." In M. A. Bayne Smith (ed.), *Race, Gender, and Health.* Thousand Oaks, Calif.: Sage, 1996.

Merton, R. K. *Social Theory and Social Structure.* New York: Free Press, 1957.

New York City Department of City Planning. *The Newest New Yorkers, 1990–1994.* New York: Department of City Planning, 1996.

Remine, D., Rice, R. M., and Ross, J. *Self-Help Groups and Human Service Agencies: How They Work Together.* New York: Family Service of America, 1984.

Rubin, H. J., and Rubin, I. S. *Community Organizing and Development.* (2nd ed.) Boston: Allyn & Bacon, 1992.

Salamon, L. M. (ed.). *Beyond Privatization: The Tools of Government Action.* Washington, D.C.: Urban Institute Press, 1989.

Salamon, L. M. "The Crisis of the Nonprofit Sector and the Challenge of Renewal." *National Civic Review,* 1996, *85*(4), 3–16.

Sampson, C. C. "Health Care Problems in the 1980s from a Black Perspective." *Journal of the National Medical Association,* 1984, *76,* 968–971.

Schlesinger, M. "Paying the Price for Medical Care: Minorities and the Newly Competitive Health Care System." *Milbank Quarterly,* 1987, *65,* 270–296.

Shannon, T. R., Kleniewski, N., and Cross, W. M. *Urban Problems in Sociological Perspective.* (3rd ed.) Prospect Heights, Ill.: Waveland Press, 1997.

Swarns, R. L. "'African American' Becomes a Term for Debate." *New York Times,* Aug. 29, 2004, p. 1.

Warren, R. L. *Studying Your Community.* New York: Free Press, 1965.

Watson, K., and Gold, S. D. *The Other Side of Devolution: Shifting Relationships Between State and Local Governments.* Washington, D.C.: Urban Institute Press, 1997.

Winn, M. "Competitive Health Care: Assessing an Alternative Solution for Health Care Problems." In W. Jones Jr. and M. F. Rice (eds.), *Health Care Issues in Black America: Policies, Problems, and Prospects.* Westport, Conn.: Greenwood Press, 1987.

Planning for Sustainability

Yvonne J. Graham

Over the past two decades, mainstream health care services in the United States have moved in the direction of primary prevention, an area in which CBHOs have consistently been at the forefront. Consequently, CBHOs are increasingly sought out as essential partners in health service planning and delivery because of their capacity not only to reach but also to penetrate underserved communities. Although they are gaining national recognition for their important role, they face constant threats to their sustainability. This is in large part due to the fact that there is a dearth of research documenting their effectiveness as well as lack of long-term investments in this particular genre of health service delivery.

As we go forward, there is also a need for CBHOs to build their capacity and position themselves to grow and compete with market forces. To do so, they will have to conduct more rigorous assessment, evaluation, documentation, and dissemination of the work they do.

Evaluation is of particular importance because it is a means of providing evidence-based justification that speaks to the quality and effectiveness of the significant work being done by CBHOs.

Learning Objectives

- Heavy reliance on government support, a more restrictive health care financial environment, and market competition threaten the survival of CBHOs.

- There is increasing evidence that CBHOs are essential partners in the delivery of health services and have the ability to
  reach underserved and culturally diverse populations in a way
  that mainstream systems cannot.
- Because of the important role they play, CBHOs must increase
  their chances of survival by engaging in strategic capacity-
  building initiatives to ensure growth and sustainability.
- CBHOs must evaluate their programs and services in order
  to amass the kinds of data that will provide evidence of what
  strategies are effective, how they were implemented, and what
  makes the CBHO approach a successful format for improving
  health outcomes.

Evolutionary Forces: Demand Versus Capacity

This chapter is devoted to describing the importance of planning
as a tool for strengthening the capacity of community-based health
organizations (CBHOs) to effectively deliver services to their constituents. It will also present a number of strategies and guidelines
that can assist CBHOs in setting the stage for organizational sustainability and growth.

The context and content of this chapter follow information on
CBHO research provided in Chapter Three and the case study of the
Caribbean Women's Health Association in Chapter Four. Additional
information was gleaned from a study on New York City's nonprofit
sector conducted by the New York City Nonprofit Project (Seley and
Wolpert, 2002) and a six-month study of community-based AIDS organizations conducted by the Center for an Urban Future (2003).

An examination of all these sources found a number of similarities in the mission, structure, and function of CBHOs, and all
of the studies validated the importance of CBHOs in providing
neighborhood-based, culturally sensitive services to underserved
populations. There were also striking similarities in the current
market position of CBHOs, the challenges they face, and their outlook for the future.

The majority of CBHOs reported a number of internal problems that affect their ability to provide needed services to their constituents, both in the short and long term, painting a bleak outlook
for long-term sustainability. Among them are these:

- Excessive dependence on government funding, with resulting pitfalls such as low overhead support, no increases in funding in the face of increasing program costs, discontinuation of programs, and bureaucratic delays in reimbursement for services rendered
- Limited administrative support to engage in capacity-building initiatives to enable their organizations to enhance service delivery, compete successfully in the market place, attract new funding, and grow
- Inability to offer employees competitive salaries and benefits, resulting in high staff turnover rates

Externally, as the health care financial environment becomes increasingly restrictive, large institutions, in an effort to secure market share, are vying for the same funds that were traditionally given to CBHOs, particularly for community outreach services. This has put many CBHOs out of business (Bayne Smith and Perot, 2003), as they are often unable to compete successfully with these larger institutions. The CHBOs that do survive are operating under such severe financial constraints and capacity-building restrictions that their sustainability is uncertain.

Ironically, at the same time, there is increasing evidence pointing to the importance of CBHOs in the delivery of community health services and in reaching underserved populations in a way that mainstream services cannot. The Center for an Urban Future (2003), in a report on New York City's response to the AIDS crisis, argues that CBHOs, by virtue of their understanding of the communities they serve, are better able to provide comprehensive services and tend to take innovative approaches to respond to their particular needs.

At the 1999 conference "Neighborhood Health Partnerships: Building a Strong Future," designed by the Academy for Educational Development's Center for Community-Based Health Strategies for the Annie E. Casey Foundation, the participating CBHOs validated the essential role that CBHOs play in serving as a base of support and adjustment for new immigrants and as a point of entry into the health care and social service system. In fact, CBHOs often serve as the only source of health care for many individuals (Anderson, Hoffman, and Davidson, 1999). This is particularly true in predominantly immigrant communities. Factors such as differences in language, culture, pattern of health service use, and immigration issues often lead them to neighborhood-based CBHOs, where they feel a sense of cultural connection and trust (Leicher, 2001).

Because of the essential role CBHOs play as partners in the spectrum of health care delivery, there is a crucial need to reverse this trend of increasing organizational fragility. There are many lessons to be learned from high-performance corporate firms that have reengineered their businesses to maintain competitive advantages through strategies such as investing in the right people, providing high-quality services, finding and developing their market niche, engaging in strategic and operational planning, diversifying strategies, and building strategic alliances (Harrigan, 1993).

An article in the *IBM Systems Journal* put it succinctly: "To compete in today's changing competitive environment, new strategic responses are required" (Boynton, Victor, and Pine, 1993, p. 40). The fundamental pillars of these redesign strategies for CBHOs are anchored in effective planning, with the objective of developing strong internal controls, enhancing service delivery, cultivating strong external relationships, and building organizational resources.

This is by no means an easy task for already stretched organizations with administratively thin staffing structures. Both planning and capacity building require significant human, material, and financial investment. But they are the most realistic and targeted avenues for laying the groundwork for building organizational capacity to sustain long-term growth.

Planning: An Essential Tool in Organizational Capacity Building

The single most important tool in building organizational capacity is planning. The ultimate goal of planning is to enable an organization to effectively and efficiently deliver services to a particular population, to survive in a climate of constant change and stringent economic and market forces, and to grow. Planning provides the opportunity for the organization to accomplish several tasks:

• Review its history, purpose, philosophy, target population, service area, and programs on a regular basis

- Develop systematic procedures to ensure the most effective use of available resources
- Create, implement, and measure objectives that will achieve desired outcomes and facilitate future growth and sustainability
- Maintain a balance of specific strategic actions for short-term efficiency and long-term adaptability

There are three major elements in the planning process: strategic or long-range planning, operational or short-term planning, and performance monitoring. These will be described in more detail in this chapter.

As CHBOs attempt to build organizational capacity and move from their current state to a future desired state, they must anticipate and plan for the many challenges inherent in this transition. During this transformation, the organization must address external as well as internal factors that will influence its ability to move into the future. Although this transition period can be turbulent, an understanding of the dynamics of change can reduce many of the problems associated with the change process that interfere with planning.

This argument is supported by a highly respected model that describes how successful companies deal with innovation and change, in which the authors postulate that at different stages in their evolution, organizations will respond differently, depending on internal and external influences (Abernathy and Utterback, 1998). This means that the persons involved in the process of planning, in which there is inherent change, need a great deal of flexibility to adapt to internal and external evolutionary stimuli.

Examples of these evolutionary forces are technological progress, globalization, market forces, and trends in health care, all of which create uncertainties for the future and make planning difficult. Therefore, contingencies for uncontrollable factors that may have an impact on the organization must be built into the planning process. For CBHOs, these may include discontinuation of government support, population changes due to increasing cultural diversity, emerging public health and environmental issues, health care and immigration reform, and changes in political representation.

Among the most frequently used strategies in contingency planning for CHBOs are setting aside reserves to cover unexpected costs, diversifying of funding sources to ensure continued service, building resources and alliances, and developing an alternative plan for maintaining or streamlining the workforce (Anderson, Hoffman, and Davidson, 1999).

Planning involves change, and people by nature tend to resist change. Resistance may be motivated by fear of a disruption in the familiar way of doing things, uncertainties about the future, or a perceived threat to personal power and control. Regardless of the reason, people will be more comfortable and more committed if they understand the reason for the change and are allowed to have a stake in the process through participation and feedback. In *What Works for Me,* Thomas Horton (1986) identifies certain qualities and competencies of successful CEOs. Among the competencies needed by leaders who are responsible for engineering change are the following:

- The ability to identify potential points of resistance and set clear expectations in an atmosphere of open communication
- The ability to communicate a clear image of the future, articulating the benefits and costs of change
- The ability to encourage dialogue, education, personal involvement, and peer support of all members of the organization in the change process
- The ability to provide hands-on leadership to support the change process
- The ability to develop feedback mechanisms to monitor progress and generate enthusiasm in the change process

Planning also requires the involvement of managers and in many cases all individuals in the organization. Many managers do not like to plan. Planning is a continual activity; it takes time and thought, and it is hard work because policies, procedures, and systems are being altered. This can be overwhelming in organizations with an administratively thin staff. Encouraging managers to use innovation and creativity to come up with alternative approaches to attain the objectives is one way to develop a positive attitude toward planning. However, alternative approaches should be cost-effective and have the probability of success.

Another way to encourage participation is through the hands-on involvement of top-level executives. This sends a clear message of organizationwide involvement and commitment and generates enthusiasm. In addition, interdepartmental and interprogram collaboration fosters the sharing of collective ideas and best practices and ensures that the objectives and actions of the different parts of the organization are consistent with the organization's thrust.

Many CBHOs lack the technical skills to engage in formal planning. But the importance of planning as a vehicle for sustainability and growth mandates that CBHOs become vigorous in harnessing resources to support their planning efforts. The board of directors is often an untapped reservoir of talent. In addition, technical assistance is often available through funders, membership organizations, and foundations. Building strategic alliances is an excellent means of accessing information and sharing resources.

CBHOs should exercise caution when receiving technical assistance from individuals such as consultants who are not connected with the organization. Although they can provide excellent examples of best practices and pitfalls to avoid from their experience working with other organizations, ongoing involvement of persons within the organization is crucial in ensuring that the consultants' plan is consistent with the mission, goals, and objectives of the organization.

Organizational Assessment

In today's climate of technological advances, increased market competition, economic constraints, and continuous change, CBHOs are challenged to take bold steps to strengthen their capacity to not only continue to deliver services but also grow and sustain themselves. Before embarking on any undertaking to build organizational capacity, the stakeholders must have a good understanding of how the organization is functioning, of what works and what does not work. This can be accomplished by conducting an assessment of the organization's current situation.

The value of an organizational assessment is that it presents a clear picture of how the organization operates, the resources it currently has and what it needs, its market position, and its market niche. It also provides insights into factors that affect the organization's ability to deliver existing services, attract new funding, and grow. Finally, it serves as a strong basis for making decisions about the direction in which the organization should go and as a framework for developing strategies and concrete action steps to advance the organization's mission (Beadle de Palomo and Luna, 1999).

The first step in organizational assessment is to gather a small team charged with this responsibility. Technical experts and local talent may be sought to work closely with the board of directors and executive staff to carry out this task. Organizational assessment involves examining the internal and external environment. Internal assessment includes taking an inventory of the organization's programs and services, resources, strengths and weaknesses, opportunities, and threats. External assessment focuses on the population to be served, service needs, available resources, the economic, social, and political climate, and competitive forces that may affect the organization's ability to maintain service levels (Beadle de Palomo and Luna, 1999).

Figure 6.1 illustrates the essential elements in organizational assessment and planning. The narrative that follows is a prototype that can serve as a guide for benchmarking and strengthening the relevant areas of organizational functioning. It includes some of the elements illustrated in the figure.

Assessing the Internal Environment

To assist in assessing the internal environment, the following questions are useful.

What Is the Vision of the Organization? The organization's vision is a picture of what the organization will be like at a given time in the future (Beadle de Palomo and Luna, 2000). The vision combines the history of the organization with its current position and projections for the future to create an image toward which people can aspire. The vision defines the organization broadly in terms of its mission, programs, community status, and relationships with stakeholders. The board of directors and key employees develop it.

Central to the development of a vision is the principle of community participation and empowerment (Kreuter, Lezin, Kreuter, and Green, 2003). Lawrence Green and Marshall Kreuter have long emphasized and advanced the concept that consistent community involvement is a requirement for full adoption and ownership of a vision for improved health not only from residents but also from all stakeholders, which then ensures that the resulting

Figure 6.1. Elements in
Organizational Assessment and Planning.

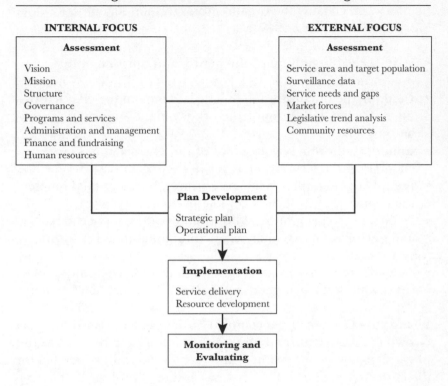

interventions will be effective. These concepts have provided the basis on which several large-scale national projects were developed at the community level (Green and Kreuter, 1990; Kreuter, 1992). A broad vision designed with community input that describes where the organization wants to be at some future point makes it possible to develop a focused mission statement.

Is the Mission Statement Consistent with Current and Future Goals? The mission statement describes why the organization exists, the goals and outcomes it seeks to achieve, and whom it serves. Writing it out ensures clarity of purpose and consistency, internally and externally, and serves as a focus for all major planning decisions. The mission statement defines the general course and goal priorities for the organization and guides the activities of leaders and employees. The mission statement should be reviewed periodically and revised as necessary. The following guidelines are helpful when creating the organization's mission statement (Below, Morrisey, and Acomb, 1987):

- Write a clear definition of the nature and purpose of the organization.
- Describe the organization's "niche" or any unique characteristic that makes it different from other organizations doing similar business.
- Conduct a thorough assessment of the organization's current clientele and review any changes in the recent past.
- Identify demographic or migration trends that might change the characteristics of the clientele in the future.
- Delineate the geographical boundaries of the service area, and perform a needs analysis of contiguous areas for future consideration.
- Analyze the kinds of services the organization currently provides, and perform a needs analysis for potential new services.

What Is the Current Organizational Structure, and Can It Support Growth? The structure of an organization can be defined as the physical, material, professional, and technical resources needed for the entity to operate and the systems and relationships that are required for efficient and effective functioning. An organization chart showing hierarchy, lines of communication, and relationships inside and outside the organization, accompanied by job descriptions outlining roles and responsibilities and by operating policies and procedures, can give a quick snapshot of the structure of the CBHO.

However, the critical issue is to determine whether this structure is adequately supporting the functions of the organization. Can that structure accommodate growth, and if not, what structures are needed now and in the future? To answer these questions, it is important to understand some of the issues around the evolution and structural development of CBHOs.

First, many CBHOs, especially those serving immigrant populations, struggle to provide services with minimal staff, driven by their sense of commitment as well as demand for their expertise and thus caught in the quandary of supply and demand.

Second, CBHOs often seek funding either because it is available or because there is a demand for the services. In many cases, the funding is not sufficient to cover the full cost of the program, and the organization is not in a position to make up the difference. In an effort to meet the needs of their constituents or because of grant restrictions, they expend the majority of funds on front-line staff, leaving the organization too administratively thin to adequately manage its operations and grow.

Based on these factors, in examining the organizational structure, an inventory of current professional and technical skills as well as material and physical resources, systems, and relationships is an essential tool. The findings should then be measured against what is ideally needed for the successful operation of the organization now and in the next three to five years.

Because of funding limitations to build capacity, combined with market forces, many CBHOs that traditionally operated as independent entities are now exploring a variety of partnership arrangements with other community organizations such as religious institutions, schools, hospitals, and clinics. These models will be discussed in greater detail in Chapter Seven.

Can the Board of Directors Provide the Leadership Necessary for Organizational Development and Financial Growth? One of the biggest challenges for CBHOs is to assemble a board of directors that is committed, active, and able to raise funds to maintain and grow the organization. Individuals who agree to volunteer their time and resources as board members want to be of assistance. But too often they are not asked to participate in a meaningful way. The key to success in creating an effective and committed board lies in strong leadership, harnessing the creative talents and technical skills of board members, selecting individuals who can advance the mission and goals of the organization, providing opportunities for training and development, building relationships and trust, and keeping the board members active and informed (Honig, 1988).

While board members may perform different tasks according to their interest or expertise, all should participate in fundraising. Their participation can be on different levels according to their skills and availability. For example, some members may be the spokespersons for the organization, participating in activities such as radio and television interviews or cultivating relationships with potential funders. Others can assist with grant writing, event planning, or mail campaigns and follow-up.

An important fundraising strategy is for board members to donate to the organization. This is in keeping with the old adage that "charity begins at home." When board members give, it sends a message to potential donors that they care, that they are making an investment, and so can the prospective donor. In fact, active and involved board members impress many funders. Remember, enthusiasm is contagious.

Are Financial Systems Adequate? One of the key pillars of organizational sustainability is good financial management. This includes having systems in place that can effectively manage current funding and support financial growth and also having in place strong administrative systems to monitor compliance with policies and procedures (Caribbean Women's Health Association, 2002). It is the responsibility of the board of directors to ensure that the organization has the appropriate internal financial control and administrative systems for proper accounting, management, and reporting.

Financial controls include the following:

- Proper accounting procedures
- Accuracy of accounts and appropriate classification of funds
- Appropriate cost control measures
- Appropriate monitoring of accounting records
- Security of assets

Administrative controls include the following:

- Accounting policies to provide guidelines on the accounting and administration of grants
- Internal control policies to ensure that the business is conducted in an ethical manner and that the organization's assets are safeguarded
- Cost accounting policies to provide guidelines in cost allocation particularly for multiple programs
- Compensation policies related to fringe benefits, consultants, and other expenditures of funds

- Property management policies to ensure proper disposition of property, equipment, and materials
- Policies to account for the organization's assets, liabilities, and fund balance

Additional Areas of Internal Assessment

In addition to answering the questions just cited, planning and assessment of the internal environment must also focus on two other important areas: administration and management, and human resources.

Administration and Management.   The overall objective of the CBHO is to serve people, and the primary goal of management is to move the organization toward accomplishing this objective. Effective management includes the personal management skills, systems, and policies needed for the organization to function well. The effective manager should have good organizational and planning skills, leadership and motivational abilities, good social and communication skills, and public health competencies. The systems and policies needed include strategic and operational plans, strong internal controls, human resource development, fund development, marketing and communications, relationship building, and evaluation mechanisms. In addition, adequate and safe facilities for administrative and program activities are basic requirements for an organization to operate efficiently.

Kuhl (1977) describes a set of management practices that are needed for the effective functioning of health service organizations and can be applied to CBHOs, including the following:

- Ensuring that all employees fully understand how responsibilities are divided among individuals and departments
- Developing communication patterns and reporting systems
- Engaging in planning activities
- Effectively allocating human and financial resources
- Working cooperatively with the board of directors to provide adequate salary and fringe benefits for employees
- Ensuring ongoing staff development and training
- Developing and improving technological systems

- Building strong internal financial control systems
- Improving the quality and accessibility of services through ongoing evaluation and quality control mechanisms
- Increasing the organization's visibility and promoting its programs and services
- Influencing legislation through advocacy

Human Resources. Getting the right people for the job and keeping them is one of the everyday challenges many CBHOs face. The right people are those with the necessary professional skills, experience, and commitment to carry out the mandates of the organization. In his book *Jack: Straight from the Gut* (2001), Jack Welch, former CEO of General Electric, underscores the importance of getting the right people. For him, he said, "it made all the difference in the world" (p. 53).

Chapter Four highlights the professional competencies that enhance the ability of CBHO employees to work with culturally diverse populations. These competencies revolve around knowledge of the target population and their service needs, understanding of the social and political environment of the community and their impact on the organization's ability to deliver services, and the ability to foster trust and collaboration between clients, community institutions, government agencies, and funders (Windsor, Baranowski, Clark, and Cutter, 1984).

Although many employees are committed to the mission and goals of CBHOs, retaining employees is an ongoing problem. Budgetary constraints and grant restrictions limit the ability of CBHOs to increase salaries, offer competitive rates, or provide attractive benefits. Focus group discussions with nonprofit leaders revealed that nonprofits had difficulty recruiting staff and were losing valuable employees to the private sector and government (Seley and Wolpert, 2002). Uncertainty about long-term support from government threatens the stability of programs. Furthermore, chronic cash flow problems experienced by CBHOs often result in late payrolls and contribute to low morale, low productivity, and ultimately the loss of valuable employees.

Key strategies in recruiting and retaining CBHO employees include the following:

- Foster a sense of ownership in the organization and the community by involving employees in decision making and inviting their creativity in improving the organization. Ownership in this context is best described as "when everybody depends on everybody else, when there are sponsors rather than bosses, and when objectives are set by those who must make them happen" (Peters and Austin, 1985, p. 233).
- Provide clear channels of communication that keep employees abreast of successes and accomplishments as well as opportunities and threats.
- Provide opportunities for personal and professional development.
- Maintain an employee recognition program in which employees are rewarded for a job well done.

In addition to solid strategies for recruiting and retaining quality staff, ongoing monitoring of performance is indispensable. A critical question to be answered periodically to assess the fit among staff, services, and client need is, Are programs and services meeting the needs of the target population? It is important to periodically take an inventory of the population being served by the program. This is of particular relevance in urban areas where there is constant population movement resulting from immigration and economic forces. The population may be defined by race, ethnicity, age range, gender, language, income, immigrant status, or any combination thereof.

The next step is to obtain and analyze information on the current status of that population to determine what needs there are, what resources currently exist to address those needs, the appropriateness or effectiveness of those services, and service gaps. This information can be collected in periodic client interviews and surveys or through more formal needs assessment. Client feedback must be obtained, as it is very useful in describing and prioritizing service needs, developing appropriate interventions, avoiding duplication in services, and setting the stage for collaboration with existing community resources.

The types of services to be offered by the organization should be consistent with the mission of the organization, the needs of the target population, funding availability, and adequate staffing levels with expertise to manage and operate the program. There should be justifiable reasons for continuing the current program and a clear need for adding new programs. Justification of current or new programs should show that they meet the needs of the target population and reflect the goals and priorities of the organization, that the organization has the physical and human resources for effective administration, and that the program has sufficient funding to cover all the associated costs.

Other considerations should include the potential for the program to grow, withstand market pressures, and sustain itself if funding is discontinued. This is of critical importance when different programs contribute to the overhead costs of the organization, because if one program is discontinued, it will affect the overall organization. In addition, programs or projects that have a short life span should be able to cover all their costs independently of other programs so that when they are discontinued, the overall operation is not affected.

The next determination is concerned with the service modalities, strategies, and interventions that will work best with the target population to achieve the desired program results. Service modalities and interventions typically used by CBHOs include awareness outreach, information and referral, health education, counseling, case management, and clinical care.

In making decisions about the selection of modalities and interventions, elements to consider are staffing levels and skills that will be required, the cost of implementing the interventions versus funding availability, and the data that will be required for evaluation of program quality and effectiveness.

Assessing the External Environment

The organization's external environment typically refers to the population it serves, the geographical boundaries of the service area, and the structures within those boundaries. The external environment extends beyond those boundaries, however, to include other individuals, geographical areas, and institutions that are connected with the organization, its clients, and its services. Examples are legislators and policymakers, funding sources and government institutions, and clients' country of origin in the case of immigrants.

Assessment of the external environment provides information about how the organization relates to its external environment. It also identifies the market position of the organization with respect to its programs and services, competitors, opportunities, and challenges. Environmental assessment may take many forms, depending on the depth of information needed or the purpose for which it will be used (Beadle de Palomo and Luna, 2000). For example, if a new service is to be introduced, it is prudent to obtain information on the demographic, socioeconomic, and cultural characteristics and health indicators of the population to be served. A study of the geographical boundaries and the structures and resources within those communities will also be important in determining service gaps, to avoid duplication of efforts, and for coordinating purposes. Equally important is the need to understand the political and market dynamics of the community.

Similarly, for fundraising purposes, assessing the organization's knowledge of and relationship with businesses, corporations, community leaders, potential funders, clients, and other appropriate individuals can be incorporated into fundraising initiatives.

Strategic Planning

Literature on strategic planning as an organizational development tool is extensive. Strategic planning is a conceptualization of where an organization intends to be in the future and how it will get there. It focuses on long-term results. Although the time frame will depend on the purpose of the organization, in the nonprofit world it is typically a three- or five-year period. The strategic plan is not a document to be left on a shelf. It is a blueprint that will guide the development and implementation of specific objectives to achieve the goals outlined in it. The strategic plan must be revisited frequently to determine level of goal achievement. It may also be revised before its "expiration date" to reflect changes in the organization's internal or external environment.

The overall objective of the strategic plan is to strengthen the ability of the organization to deliver appropriate and quality services to its clients. Strategic planning affects or involves everyone connected with the organization in some way. Accordingly, the leaders and employees have important roles involving critical choices and priority setting. The needs and expectations of clients are important in determining the types and levels of programs to be offered. Community leaders and institutions are essential to program intervention, coordinating, and resource-building and advocacy efforts.

The strategic planning process involves many people. It is sometimes carried out in small teams that include representatives from the organization's board of directors, top executives, various levels of staff, members of the client population, and in some cases, consultants and technical experts who actually develop the plan. Among the various categories of participants in this process, consultants tend not to have a stake in the organization. Therefore, the active involvement of members of the organization and the community being served is crucial when making decisions about choices and strategy development.

The strategic planning process begins with a needs assessment, described earlier in this chapter. The needs assessment reveals the current situation of the organization, including its purpose and functions, programs and service mix, service delivery approach, client base and identified needs, its constituency base, and its successes and challenges. Information gathered from the needs assessment, combined with a shared vision, forms the basis on which key issues are identified and priorities are set. The priorities are then translated into goals.

The body of knowledge required for developing the strategic plan comes from the needs assessment and should provide the answer to the following questions:

- What kind of business is the organization identified by, whom does it serve, and what is the uniqueness of its services? For example, the organization may exist to provide health education services, and its uniqueness may be the provision of services to immigrants from a particular country.
- What are the operating beliefs, practices, and policy principles of the organization? These revolve around a set of core values, a philosophy, and practices that demonstrate those core values and that philosophy. These elements form the foundation for the organization's image, culture, and modus operandi.
- What is the current mix of programs and services, and is there a likelihood that these services will be in demand in the fu-

ture? The mix of programs will be influenced by health care trends, emerging health issues, demographic shifts, and competitive forces.

- What is the current performance in terms of financial and human resources, client outcomes, and service delivery mechanisms?
- What are the successes and challenges, strengths and weaknesses of the organization? How can the successes and strengths be developed into "core competencies" and marketed as "best practices"?
- What do the stakeholders want the organization to look like in three to five years?
- What resources will be needed to help it get there, and is the organization capable of providing those resources? If not, what are the alternatives?
- What are the major weaknesses that might impede progress?
- What steps should be taken to address these weaknesses and plan for growth?
- What external changes could have an impact on the organization's ability to accomplish its goals?
- What contingencies should be put in place to address those uncontrollable external factors?

Operational Planning

The operational plan is an action tool for systematically mapping out the tasks and resources needed to achieve the goals and priorities of the strategic plan. Whereas the strategic plan is conceptual, focused on broad goals and the long term, the operational plan is results-oriented, focused on tasks to be accomplished within a specific time frame. For most CBHOs, the time frame is one year. Since the goals of the strategic plan are to be accomplished over the longer term, the board of directors and executive team make a determination about which key issues and goals from the strategic plan should be prioritized in terms of time and importance.

Every manager in the organization must be involved in developing the operational plan so that efforts in each area of responsibility all contribute to the organizationwide plan. Below, Morrisey, and Acomb (1987) provide some guidelines on operational planning from which the following key guidelines were formed:

- Determine the objectives to be achieved within the year, focusing on those with the potential for success.
- Delineate specific action steps to be taken in order to attain those objectives.
- Determine the human, material, and financial resources that will be needed to implement the action steps, and clearly establish how personnel will be deployed.
- Establish deadlines for the achievement of objectives with built-in interim monitoring schedules.
- Establish criteria and determine the tools and mechanisms to measure the attainment of the objectives.

To maintain interest and enthusiasm in executing the operational plan, particularly when people are apprehensive about change, it is advisable that organizations focus initially on strategies that are achievable and have the potential for success. Rudolph W. Giuliani, the former mayor of New York City, in his book *Leadership* (2002) provides some excellent case studies about small successes and their value in boosting the morale.

Performance Monitoring

Part of the execution of the operational plan is to monitor progress along the way. This is critical in reducing risks especially in new ventures or approaches. It is also helpful in identifying problems, needs, opportunities, and threats while tasks are being implemented so that appropriate action can be taken. Finally, it provides an opportunity for feedback and input from employees.

Strategies for Sustainability

Reliance on government support, continued low funding, and repeated assaults by budget cuts have resulted in increasing fragility for CBHOs. To reverse this trend, CBHOs must develop strategies and implement activities that will build their capacity to continue to provide services, sustain themselves, and grow. Among the most realistic and targeted avenues for laying this groundwork are diversifying funding streams, building strategic alliances, and strengthening organizational infrastructure.

Diversifying the Funding Streams

This chapter at the outset identified financial woes as the number one threat to the survival of CBHOs. It took special note of the heavy reliance on government funding, uncertainties about level of support and continuity, chronic cash flow problems, and lack of capacity to attract new funding required for organizational maintenance and growth.

Diversifying the funding base by engaging in a variety of fundraising activities is one of the best ways to reduce CBHOs' reliance on government support and move toward self-sufficiency. Successful fundraising is a daunting task that takes time and human investment. It involves a number of developmental steps to prepare the organization to effectively market its services and manage growth. These include strengthening the organization's internal financial control mechanisms, building the organization's reputation, and developing and implementing a targeted strategic fundraising plan. These are monumental tasks for fragile CBHOs that are already overburdened, strapped for cash, and understaffed. Hence the fundraising plan should be carefully thought out and should focus on objectives that are attainable, based on the organization's strengths, and will generate the most revenue.

Preparing for Fundraising: Strengthening Internal Systems

An important part of fundraising is having adequate systems in place that will convince potential donors that the organization is able to manage the funds raised and support growth. It is the responsibility of the board of directors and management to ensure that appropriate internal financial and administrative controls are in place for proper accounting, monitoring, and reporting.

Funders often request financial information as part of the grant application process. This may take the form of written information about financial performance and supporting documents. The following documents that provide financial information should therefore be compiled:

- Audited financial statements
- Annual reports
- Cash flow statements and balance sheet

- Financial policies and procedures
- Qualifications of personnel

In addition to strengthening the internal financial systems, CBHOs should build the organization's reputation. This means providing the highest level of commitment and service to clients and truly meeting their needs. Funders want to be associated with organizations that provide effective services. Building reputation also means increasing the organization's visibility by promoting its image, programs and services, and market niche and highlighting its leadership, successes, and accomplishments.

Cultivating Relationships with Potential Funders

Cultivating relationships with potential funders is another key developmental step in successful fundraising. These relationships help funders know about the organization and its leadership, mission, services, and funding needs. It will give funders the confidence that the organization is well suited to administer their grants or donations. Funders also want to know that their money will be well spent and that there will be accountability (Caesar & Washburn, 2001).

Targets for relationship building should include businesses that are related in some way with the organization. For example, an organization whose mission is to provide health and social services to underserved immigrant women from the Caribbean living in Brooklyn might want to seek out funders interested in ethnic groups, women, health-related organizations such as managed care companies, companies that do business with the Caribbean, and companies committed to Brooklyn.

Assessing the Marketplace

The next step in preparing for fundraising is to take an inventory of how the organization is perceived by potential funders, community residents, and community leaders and what the potential sources of funding might be. All of this information will be used to develop strategies that will best market the services of the organization. The following is a prototype of a marketing strategy and fundraising plan that can serve as a guide for CBHOs in their fundraising efforts. The plan was created for a Brooklyn-based CBHO, the Caribbean Women's Health Association, Inc. (CWHA), which was featured in Chapter Four, by the consulting firm of Caesar & Washburn, Inc. (C&W). CWHA provides health, immigration, and social support services to a predominantly immigrant population. The aim of the marketing and fundraising effort was to position the organization in the private sector funding arena and to increase its ability to raise support from that sector.

The consultants began with an internal assessment of the organization's functioning: its governance, programs, past fundraising efforts, and market position. As part of this process, C&W interviewed individuals identified as knowledgeable about the target population, their service needs, and the programs and services offered by CWHA. They also interviewed program officers at several leading foundations about issues addressed by CWHA, their priority in the marketplace, and the possibilities for philanthropic support. Analysis of the information thus gathered highlighted the issues that CWHA had to address to position itself effectively in the funding arena.

Reputation. Interviewees indicated that CWHA enjoys a unique reputation for providing the highest level of commitment and service to its clients. The organization is thought to be knowledgeable about the community it serves and is very aggressive in pursuing its mission. Many believed that CWHA was meeting a need that no one else was meeting.

External Environment. Many interviewees felt that immigrant issues do not have a high priority among businesses or civic and philanthropic leaders, and few have specifically targeted these groups for support. All of the foundation officers suggested that increased awareness could possibly result in more funding and therefore more services to immigrants. Respondents believed that outreach, information, and referral services are critical for immigrants and ranked prevention education higher than the need for direct services.

Internal Factors. Respondents believed that CWHA did not have the infrastructure necessary to support growth and suggested that the board of directors be expanded and strengthened to include more people who are well connected and perceived as "players" in Brooklyn.

Prospects for Financial Support. Interviewees were unanimous in believing that CWHA was deserving of philanthropic support, giving such compelling reasons as "Community-based health care will be the direction for health services in the future" and "Community-based health organizations like CWHA really understand the needs of immigrants and are among the few places where professionals and nonprofessionals work well together." However, most interviewees believed that it would be difficult to attract financial support from the private sector because companies have been redefining corporate social responsibility as linking their giving to their marketing needs and interest in being profitable.

Recommendations. After reviewing CWHA's sources of support, current fundraising efforts, image, programs, and visibility, C&W concluded that because of CWHA's excellent programs, strong leadership, and unique ability to address barriers to health care and other services for immigrants, it was well positioned to become a stronger leader in the field. Accordingly, the consultants recommended that CWHA take all of the following actions:

- Rethink its marketing position in the nonprofit sector and broaden its appeal to a wider range of funders by creating a targeted marketing strategy that responds directly to the specialized interest of funders.
- Match its multifaceted programs to appropriate funding areas. Major target markets identified were foundations and corporations that fund specific program areas, locally based corporations with a vested interest in the health of the locality, and citywide corporations whose products and services are used by immigrants.
- Conduct a major education and awareness campaign to educate the philanthropic community about the needs of its constituents.
- Assume leadership and forge a coalition to launch a major education campaign that may lead to increased private sector funding.
- Constitute an active, well-connected board of directors that can provide the appropriate stewardship necessary for the organization's financial growth.

- Increase its visibility in the philanthropic and business communities and with the wider public.
- Establish a fundraising calendar that includes a foundation campaign, a corporate campaign, a recognizable major annual event, and several other cultivation and fundraising events throughout the year.

Developing the Fundraising Strategies

Based on the assessment findings and the consultants' recommendations, the following marketing strategy and fundraising plan were developed.

GOAL 1: To undertake a range of cultivation activities that can attract new friends and supporters and firmly establish the organization as a major player in the field

Cultivation Activities

- A corporate and foundation reception to introduce CWHA to potential corporate and foundation donors
- An annual breakfast seminar for businesses, funders, elected officials, health professionals, and community leaders to provide the opportunity to showcase CWHA's programs and give an update on critical issues affecting the community
- House parties in homes of board members to provide the opportunity for board members to introduce CWHA to their circle of friends and acquaintances
- Offering CWHA as a partner to corporations based on reciprocity—the value it can provide to a sponsor

GOAL 2: To establish a major annual fundraising drive, including a foundation campaign, a corporate campaign, an individual gifts program, a recognizable annual event, a direct mail campaign, and other activities

Fundraising Activities

- Foundation Campaign: Set a realistic dollar amount as the goal. Create and implement a targeted marketing approach to successfully appeal to foundation and corporate foundation givers.

- Individual Gifts Program: Set a realistic dollar amount as the goal. Have board members solicit donations from their friends and past supporters. Nurture relationship with current donors.
- Special Events: Set a realistic dollar amount as the goal. Establish a Friends Committee, and plan an annual event building on lessons learned from past events.
- Celebrity Concert: Set a realistic dollar amount as the goal. Seek one or more celebrities to do a benefit and donate part of the proceeds to the organization.
- Mail Campaign: Set a realistic dollar amount as the goal. Send out a well-constructed appeal letter to familiarize a broader base of individuals with the work of the organization and solicit contributions.

Building Strategic Alliances

Forming partnerships has become an important capacity-building and survival strategy for CBHOs. These partnerships are known by many names: *coalitions, alliances, collaboratives, consortia.* The term *partnership* usually refers to a relationship between two or more organizations, while *coalitions, collaboratives,* and *alliances* normally involve multiple organizations.

These collaborations also have a wide variety of structure and functions. Some are formed to accomplish a specific objective—most often to advocate for a particular piece of legislation or to share information about a specific issue (McKay, 2000). Others are formed to address a variety of issues relating to service delivery, research, or advocacy. Some are formed to fulfill funding requirements and others for leveraging resources, expanding market share, capitalizing on market niche, managing funds, or building organizational capacity. Partnership structures range along the spectrum from formal legal entities to loose cooperation based on available time and resources. Regardless of the reason for which they are formed, entering into partnerships and strategic alliances has become a common and almost indispensable organizational development strategy.

Literature, conferences, and workshops on the topic of coalitions, collaborations, and partnerships and their successes and challenges abound. The following outline of essential elements in building effective partnerships was gleaned from the literature and from my own experience. For uniformity of this discussion, the term *coalition* will be used.

As public funds allocated for health care become more scarce, many CBHOs are receiving smaller grant allocations or are forced to seek small grants from multiple sources. Often the grant funds received are not sufficient to provide the level of services required to address a health issue. Therefore, many CBHOs enter into collaborative arrangements with other organizations so that they can share their experiences and combine and use resources in a way that would be more beneficial to each partner than if they acted alone.

Although these efforts have been successful, they are often entered into with much apprehension because organizations fear competition for market share and market niche or fear losing their individual strengths and identity. In this context, it is important that individuals participating in coalitions have a clear understanding of the difference between collaboration and competition and are assured that their organization's identity will be preserved. Developing trust among all parties involved in the coalition is another key strategy in harmonizing people to work across organizational boundaries.

When coalitions are intended to operate over the long term, a formal structure should be put in place to provide leadership in determining the goals, priorities, membership involvement, and operation of the coalition. From the outset, there should be a shared commitment among members to work together to achieve a common goal.

To minimize conflicts, coalition members should have a clear sense of the coalition's goals and activities, the decision-making process, the results that are to be achieved, and their individual roles and responsibilities. Many coalitions are formed to apply for funding that would be distributed to each organization to implement specific activities. It is of paramount importance that participating organizations have a leadership structure in place to guide the coalition's efforts. Also, members of the coalition should agree in writing on the policies and process for distribution of economic and program resources.

Among the critical structural issues to be considered for the effective operation of the coalition are criteria for membership eligibility, a clear and preagreed decision-making process, opportunities for active participation and feedback mechanisms, and an equitable division of resources.

Constituting a Strong Board of Directors

Nonprofit organizations are typically governed by a board of directors serving in a voluntary capacity. The board of directors is responsible for making decisions about the organization's goals and resources. A strong board of directors is able to provide stable leadership, bring visibility to the organization, ensure the organization's continued ability to carry out the range of activities essential for its growth, and enable it to better respond to the needs of the population it serves.

One of the primary responsibilities of the board of directors is to develop, review, and revise the constitution and by-laws of the organization. The constitution and by-laws are among the important corporate legal documents required under not-for-profit corporate law. In addition to being a legal requirement, by-laws are specific to the mission and operation of the organization. They facilitate the smooth running of the organization and provide policies for resolving potential conflicts.

Provisions of the by-laws include the legal name of the organization, membership and composition, tenure, committees and their roles and responsibilities, conflict-of-interest policies, legal and fiduciary responsibilities, and transaction, dissolution, and indemnification clauses.

Along with the executive management, the board of directors is responsible for ensuring that the organization has the necessary licenses, accreditation, and corporate documents required by entities that serve the public through charitable, religious, cultural, or other activities. They must also adhere to the responsibilities that accompany nonprofit status, such as public accountability, financial soundness, and compliance with government regulations (Brooklyn in Touch, 1987). Among the items required to operate legally are the constitution and by-laws; articles of incorporation; federal employer identification certificate; federal, state, and local tax exemptions; nonprofit 501(c)(3) status; charities registration; and required insurance coverage.

The number of persons serving on a board varies. However, there should be enough members to work in committees to carry out the activities of the board. The most common activities in which board members are involved are policymaking, strategic planning, financial oversight, corporate and community outreach, and fundraising.

Recruiting the right mix of board members and retaining them is one of the most challenging tasks for nonprofit organizations. In order to select individuals who can best serve the organization, detailed answers to the following questions should be developed:

- Who should serve on the board?
- What level of commitment is required of board members?
- What activities are board members expected to be involved in?
- What skills and experience are required to implement those activities?

Board members are chosen for various reasons. Some funders require that a particular percentage of board members reflect characteristics of the population served with respect to race and ethnicity. Consumer representation may also be a requirement of funders. Some members are selected because of their connection with the organization, the community, or the programs and services being offered. Others are selected because of their particular expertise and their ability to connect the organization with needed resources.

Commitment to the mission and goals of the organization must be among the key criteria in selecting board members (Caribbean Women's Health Association, 2002). In general, board members should meet all of the following criteria:

- They have a genuine concern and interest in the work of the organization.
- They are willing to give the necessary time and to use their resources to advance the goals of the organization.
- They are willing to assist either directly or indirectly in the organization's fundraising efforts.
- They are willing to accept responsibility for governance of the organization and to become involved in its activities.
- They have a track record of community involvement or have experience or expertise that will contribute to the goals of the organization.

When board members with the requisite skills are recruited, they should be appropriately oriented concerning the mission, scope of services, financial performance over the past three years (or more), legal and fiduciary responsibilities, by-laws, and policies and procedures of the board and of the organization.

Board members should be asked to be involved in concrete ways. Their involvement will vary according to their time availability, area of interest, level of expertise, or ability to connect the organization with needed resources. The task of fundraising, however, should be the responsibility of all of the members, since this is one of the most critical needs of CBHOs.

A study conducted by the New York City Nonprofits Project indicated that in the 9,078 nonprofit organizations surveyed, just under 100,000 people serve as unpaid board members. Of this number, 38 percent reported that board members make individual donations, and an additional 45 percent listed fundraising assistance as a major activity (Seley and Wolpert, 2002, p. 41).

One of the major challenges for nonprofit boards is retaining board members. Board members serve on a voluntary basis, giving of their time and resources out of commitment. Therefore, they become motivated when they feel that their services advance the mission and goals of the organization. A key strategy to retain board members and maintain a high level of enthusiasm is building a good relationship between the executive director and the board and between and among members. The board should provide the executive director with strong support, and the executive director, in turn, should maintain good communication with the chair and other members (Annie E. Casey Foundation, 2000). Putting "good and welfare" on the agenda of every meeting—permitting board members to share news of births, marriages, deaths, and other personal life events—builds relationships. Serving refreshments facilitates social interaction.

In terms of effectiveness, it is advisable to limit the length of time that individuals serve on a board. However, during their active tours of duty, board members will function more effectively if they are kept abreast of activities and developments occurring with the organization. One way to maintain the flow of information to board members is through updated, state-of-the-art management information systems.

Technology has changed the way we do things in a major way. It has increased the speed at which we receive and manage information and has improved service delivery, operations, and management. In the nonprofit world, access to and use of technology has become a necessity for survival and growth, for many reasons:

- Information technology (IT) increases the organization's ability to track client data, develop reports, communicate with a broad audience, retrieve information, conduct prospect research, and participate in electronic grant application processes.
- Many funders require that grantees collect and report data electronically using a variety of database systems.
- Tools such as a Web site enhance the organization's ability to market its programs and services, do fundraising, and link with other organizations.

Via the Internet, organizations can now access information twenty-four hours a day. This has proved to be very useful in situations such as proposal development that are in most cases time-sensitive.

The problems that CBHOs face with IT development revolve around limited funding to purchase computer hardware and software, service contracts, and staff training. As the health care funding arena becomes more restrictive, many CBHOs are not receiving increased levels of funding for various programs and services. They make the decision to spend the greater part of their budget to retain personnel, with the hope of raising additional funds to cover costs associated with non-personnel-related services, such as computer hardware and software and other equipment. Very often, sufficient money to cover those costs does not materialize, and the organizations are unable to keep up.

Devising Marketing and Communication Instruments

Organizations communicate with their clients, funders, and other publics through marketing and promotional materials. This medium serves to build and solidify goodwill for the organization, increase clientele, cultivate relationships with potential donors, influence the public to make referrals to the organization, and educate the public on the organization's programs and services.

Some communication and marketing tools are cost-free. Letters to the editor, editorials, and feature stories are a few examples.

Yet even these are generally the result of ongoing communication and marketing efforts. Among the most useful marketing and promotional tool for a CBHO is the annual report. The annual report is a good mechanism for communicating with stakeholders, interest groups, funders, and the community on the activities, accomplishments, challenges, and impact of the organization and its services. It also adds credibility to the organization. Other communication and marketing instruments include the following:

Newsletters	Lettered signs
Brochures	Journal and magazine advertisements
Flyers and posters	Billboards
Stationery	Public service announcements
Bumper stickers	Press releases
Logo or emblem	Banners
T-shirts, pens, buttons, and the like	Answering machine recording

Communication and promotional instruments should be attractive, with messages that are simple and clear. They should also be in appropriate languages and at appropriate reading levels for the target audience. It is essential that words, colors, and messages be sensitive to the audience and the subject matter.

Enhancing Service Delivery

Enhancing the delivery of services involves developing suitable policies and procedures to guide the delivery of services, establishing systems and processes for effective implementation of activities, developing standards by which services can be measured for quality and quantity, and implementing systems and processes to correct deficiencies and improve the quality of services offered. The following are important indicators of effective service delivery for CBHOs (Caribbean Women's Health Association, 2002).

Clear and Concise Documentation of Case Management Activities
There should be written policies and procedures for case management, including the content of case management records. These

should be stored in a secure area and reviewed at regular intervals for completeness and appropriateness of intervention.

Documentation of Health Education and Outreach Activities

There should be written policies and procedures for implementation and documentation of outreach and education activities. Policies and procedures should show evidence of staff training and provide guidelines for outreach and education activities. Educational curricula, handout materials, data collection instruments, and evaluation materials must be approved by appropriate individuals before they are put into use.

Appropriate Management of Client Problems

The appropriateness of problem management is best determined through client satisfaction surveys. A typical survey instrument may ask clients the following questions:

- What type of services did you receive?
- Did the receptionist or intake staff treat you with respect?
- How long did you have to wait before being seen?
- Were your needs adequately addressed?
- Was the information you received clearly explained to you?
- Please rate your level of satisfaction with the services you received.
- Would you recommend the program to a friend?
- Do you have any suggestions for improving the services?

It is important to document responses to the client surveys as well as any corrective actions taken.

Proper Use and Functioning of Equipment

To get the job done in an efficient manner, it is important that employees have the necessary equipment available and that it is maintained and accounted for at all times. Taking an inventory of equipment at regular intervals will provide important information about its usefulness and condition. This is particularly helpful when budgets are being prepared, in the event that additional funds may be required to purchase or upgrade equipment.

Service contracts should be secured where necessary, and warranty information should always be close at hand to ensure that equipment is kept in good working order. Maintaining an inventory of equipment is a critical task and is a requirement of some funding sources. Equipment is also considered as part of the organization's assets; therefore, policies and procedures must be in place to govern their use and disposal. The following are some guidelines for equipment management.

- Make an annual inventory of all equipment, its location, and where each item was purchased.
- Store manufacturers' operating manuals and warranties for all equipment in a safe and accessible place.
- Provide appropriate and secure storage for all equipment.
- Maintain repair and service contracts, and keep a log of service dates.
- Train staff to use and operate equipment properly.

Adequate Facility Operations

A safe and welcoming environment for employees and clients is indispensable. Facilities should be well maintained, clean, and well lit. Abiding by the following guidelines will ensure a safe and secure facility:

- Provide clear exterior and interior signage and adequate lighting.
- Install appropriate security devices.
- Be sure the premises are in compliance with the Americans with Disabilities Act.
- Provide well-planned spaces for employees to work in with areas for privacy where required.
- Maintain adequate insurance coverage.
- Have clear policies and procedures in place for dealing with fire and other emergencies.
- Hold regularly scheduled fire and other emergency drills.
- Post an escape plan or route that all employees are aware of.
- Be sure fire extinguishers and smoke alarms are functioning properly.
- Keep first aid kits on the premises.

Evaluation: A Critical Tool for Future Organizational Growth

Evaluation serves several purposes. Among them are monitoring the quality of client services through quality control mechanisms, monitoring the performance and productivity of employees, determining the extent to which objectives are met and the impact of targeted interventions on the population served, and such activities as program planning, program enhancement, and decision making (Windsor, Baranowski, Clark, and Cutter, 1984).

Evaluation provides critical evidence that organizations can use to document and articulate the quality, quantity, and effectiveness of interventions, lessons learned, best practices, pitfalls in service delivery, and emerging needs and issues. It also provides the organization with a guide for tailoring remedial actions. When new programs and services are introduced or when an organization is undergoing change, evaluation may be used to test the effectiveness of innovations.

There are different levels of evaluation, but they all provide feedback on the overall performance of the organization. For CBHOs that receive government and other private support, the evaluation mechanisms most frequently used to fulfill contractual obligations are process, outcome, and impact measurements.

Process Evaluation

Process evaluation is intended to increase accountability, performance, and productivity. It focuses on the quality of procedures performed by program staff and the effectiveness of operating systems to ensure the attainment of management, program-specific, and organizational objectives. It also includes information about the target population, program content, materials, media, and messages (Windsor, Baranowski, Clark, and Cutter, 1984). Process evaluation depends largely on the collection and interpretation of both quantitative and qualitative data.

Collecting quantitative data involves the recording of details of activities such as outreach, education, surveys, and case management records that can be interpreted statistically. To ensure accuracy, it is necessary to establish from the outset what type of data are to be collected, why they will be collected, the tools that will be used, who will be responsible for data collection, and how the results will be analyzed, reported, and used.

Qualitative data emanate from interviews, discussions, and surveys that provide information about feelings, attitudes, and behaviors. This information provides important feedback on the caliber, acceptability, and effectiveness of the services offered. It also provides the opportunity to correct or resolve actual or potential problems relating to the delivery of services.

To ensure the provision of safe, high-quality care and continuously improve service delivery, quality assurance activities should be a central goal of CBHOs. The purpose of quality assurance measures are as follows:

- To provide a mechanism whereby client services can be systematically reviewed to ensure quality and consistency.
- To monitor selected activities to ensure that optimal intervention is provided to avoid problems that reduce the quality of client care. These are activities that identify and document known or suspected problems and opportunities to improve services.
- To assess specific areas or functions of administration and services, including reviews of documentation, client services, equipment and supplies inventories, materials management, management information systems, security and safety, and accessibility of services.
- To administer and analyze client satisfaction tools to monitor clients' understanding of and satisfaction with the services provided.
- To ensure that problems are resolved appropriately.

Outcome Evaluation

Outcome evaluation provides information about changes in the behavior, lifestyle, or health status of the target population served. It focuses on data collection and analysis to make the connection between previous health behaviors or disease patterns, the type of program intervention, and the extent to which behavior has changed or not changed following the intervention. Outcome evaluation provides the answers to questions relating to the ability of the program to reach the individuals it intended to serve and the extent to which the interventions achieved the desired outcomes (Annie E. Casey Foundation, 2000).

Impact Evaluation

Impact evaluation is concerned with the overall ability of the organization to have a positive effect on individuals, the community, and the discipline. Broadly, it provides information about the extent to which the objectives of the strategic and operational plans are met. More specifically, it assesses the qualitative and quantitative performance of individuals, departments, programs, and services.

Conclusion

The information presented in this chapter reflects the experiences of CBHOs as defined in Chapter One. Many of these organizations evolved out of the need to respond to the needs of new immigrants and of low-income and underserved populations. There is currently a dearth of documentation on the development and infrastructural challenges these organizations face. Thus the information presented here could offer some direction for organizational development, future thought, and research.

Key Points

- CBHOs must carefully assess their internal and external environments in order to properly plan for current operations and future growth.
- Planning has to occur on four major levels—strategic, operational, results monitoring, and benchmarking—and on a variety of sublevels.
- The operating environment of CBHOs is subject to sudden and unpredictable changes. Long-term sustainability demands that CBHOs diversify their sources of funding to protect themselves from unexpected disturbances.
- Sustainability requires the building of strategic alliances and coalitions.

- One of the most reliable alliances a CBHO can develop is its board of directors. Any effort spent in building a strong board yields multiple benefits for the organization.
- Modern tools of communication and information management enhance service delivery.
- Evaluation is as important as planning. Evaluation provides the evidence of work well done and can be used to enhance the organization's image, increase its funding, and boost its long-term sustainability.

Study Questions

1. You have been called in as a consultant to assist a local CBHO in its strategic planning. Management has asked you to focus specifically on the internal environment. Compile a list of six items or documents you will ask to examine prior to taking on the assignment. Explain your rationale for asking for each of the six items or documents.
2. A group of community members is in the process of establishing a CBHO and has hired you to help constitute a strong board of directors. What criteria will you use to determine the composition or "mix" of the board, the skills required to be a board member, and the tasks board members will be asked to take on, based on their skills? Finally, what strategies will you use to retain the members once they have joined the board?

References

Anderson, M., Hoffman, R., and Davidson, S. "Neighborhood Health Partnerships: Building a Strong Future." Paper presented at the Annie E. Casey Foundation conference, Washington, D.C., 1999.

Annie E. Casey Foundation. "Building Capacity for Community Health Services: A Toolkit for Building Capacity." Conference held at the Academy for Educational Development's Center for Community-Based Health Strategies, Oct. 10–11, 2000.

Bayne Smith, M. A., and Perot, R. T. *Report of Environmental Scan of Consumer Advocacy Needs and Requirements in the District of Columbia.* Washington, D.C.: Consumer Health Foundation, 2003.

Beadle de Palomo, F., and Luna, E. *The Strategic Plan: Tools for Long-Term Planning.* Washington, D.C.: Center for Community Health Strategies, Academy for Educational Development, 2000.

Below, P. J., Morrisey, G. L., and Acomb, B. L. *The Executive Guide to Strategic Planning.* San Francisco: Jossey-Bass, 1987.

Boynton, A. C., Victor, B., and Pine, B. J., II. "New Competitive Strategies: Challenges to Organizations and Information Technology." *IBM Systems Journal,* 1993, *32,* 40–41.

Brooklyn in Touch Information Center. *How to Form and Operate a Non-Profit Corporation: Fact Sheet #2 for the Non Profit Manager.* Brooklyn, N.Y.: Brooklyn in Touch Information Center, 1987.

Caesar & Washburn. *Strategic Marketing and Fundraising Plan Developed for the Caribbean Women's Health Association.* New York: Caesar & Washburn, 2001.

Caribbean Women's Health Association. *Manual of Financial Policies and Procedures.* New York: Caribbean Women's Health Association, 2002.

Center for an Urban Future. *Epidemic Neglect: How Weak Infrastructure and Lax Planning Hinder New York City's Response to AIDS.* New York: Center for an Urban Future, 2003.

Giuliani, R. W. *Leadership: First Things First.* New York: Hyperion, 2002.

Green, L. W., and Kreuter, M. W. "Health Promotion as a Public Strategy for the 1990s." *Annual Review of Public Health,* 1990, *11,* 319–334.

Harrigan, K. R. "Issues Concerning Business-Unit and Corporate Strategy." Lecture delivered at the Columbia Business School, Executive Program in Business Administration, 1993.

Honig, L. *Evaluating Your Board of Directors.* Oakland, Calif.: Board of Directors of the *Grassroots Fundraising Journal,* 1988.

Horton, T. R. *What Works for Me: 16 CEOs Talk About Their Careers and Commitments.* New York: Random House, 1986.

Kreuter, M. W. "PATCH: Its Origin, Basic Concepts, and Links to Contemporary Public Health Policy." *Journal of Health Education,* 1992, *23,* 135–139.

Kreuter, M. W., Lezin, N. A., Kreuter, M. W., and Green, L. W. *Community Health Promotion Ideas That Work.* (2nd ed.) Boston: Jones & Bartlett, 2003.

Kuhl, I. K. *The Executive Role in Health Services Delivery Organizations.* Washington, D.C.: Office of Applied Research, Association of University Programs in Health Administration, 1977.

Leicher, S. *Voices from the Field—Building Bridges and Removing Barriers: A Strategy to Promote the Self-Sufficiency of New York's Immigrant Communities.* New York: United Way, 2001.

McKay, E. G. *Building Effective Coalitions, Collaboratives, and Consortia.* Washington, D.C.: Center for Community-Based Health Strategies, Academy for Educational Development, 2000.

Morrisey, G. L., Below, P. J., and Acomb, B. L. *The Executive Guide to Operational Planning.* San Francisco: Jossey-Bass, 1987.

Peters, T., and Austin, N. *A Passion for Excellence: The Leadership Difference.* New York: Random House, 1985.

Seley, J., and Wolpert, J. *New York City's Nonprofit Sector.* New York: New York City Nonprofits Project, 2002.

Welch, J. *Jack: Straight from the Gut.* With J. A. Byrne. New York: Warner Books, 2001.

Windsor, R. A., Baranowski, T., Clark, N. M., and Cutter, G. *Evaluation of Health Promotion and Education Programs.* Mountain View, Calif.: Mayfield, 1984.

Chapter Seven

The Future of CBHOs: Improving Health Outcomes for Everyone

Marcia Bayne Smith
Yvonne J. Graham

In this chapter, the focus is on the future of community-based health organizations (CBHOs) and their role in improving health outcomes. While there are clearly challenges ahead, there is cause for optimism and a sense of encouragement, for several reasons. First, there is every indication that CBHOs will continue to evolve and survive, as there are signs of more and more organizing going on around the country (Rivera and Erlich, 1998). Second, the various health systems in the United States continue to undergo changes as they struggle to address the multiple issues that contribute to the concentration of health disparities in specific communities and among distinct population groups (New York City Department of Health, 2004). As a result, there is an underlying perception that we are not going to be able to continue with business as usual but will instead have to adopt different approaches such as CBHOs to eliminate health disparities.

Yet the most compelling reason for optimism can be found in a renewed and invigorated interest over the past decade in improving health through community organizing and community building (Minkler and Wallerstein, 2002). One outgrowth of that interest has been the development of several models for community organizing.

Though different, the various models share a few common concepts, such as organizing for the purpose of rebuilding social capital and social cohesion and strengthening civil society (Putnam, 1996), organizing for community health education based on the principles of participation (Kreuter, 1992; Kreuter, Lezin, Kreuter, and Green, 2003), and organizing as a process of community empowerment and leadership development that ultimately leads to community change.

We know from Chapters Three and Four that CBHOs seek client participation and input to shape service delivery, including community health education, and that they advocate to create changes that will improve community health. The need at this time is for research that investigates specific CBHO contributions to rebuilding social capital and civil society and to community empowerment and leadership development.

Learning Objectives

- The most significant domestic challenge for government and health care systems in the United States is delivering primary care services to everyone in the nation in an efficient, cost-effective, culturally and linguistically appropriate manner that will serve to eliminate health disparities.
- Social and cultural changes in the country and in the health arena have already begun to yield changes in health care.
- Long-standing theoretical perspectives have begun to give way to new ways of thinking about health care delivery.
- New methods of treatment that have emerged in the past thirty years are now part of mainstream medicine.
- New research is providing evidence of greater connections between mind and body.
- Promising research methods are being developed that are more inclusive of the community, not only as research subjects but also as more active participants in the collection and analysis of data and the interpretation of results.
- The vision for the future of health care in the United States is being replicated around the world, and it includes greater emphasis on prevention, education, and wellness; greater attention to nonmedical contributing factors to premature morbidity; and a more comprehensive focus on the whole person.

- CBHOs are centrally positioned to transform health delivery by empowering communities and improving health outcomes.

The Continued Survival of CBHOs

At the start of this book, we examined the issue of community health from a historical perspective, which seems fittingly appropriate here in the final chapter. In much the same way that social and cultural changes, scientific advances, and theoretical paradigms influenced efforts to address community health problems in different ways from one era to another, they have also wrought changes in the role of health care organizations, including CBHOs.

For example, although decisions at the federal level to fund community health centers (CHCs), CBHOs, and other social programs in the 1960s and 1970s were beneficial, they did not reverse the large-scale disinvestment in poor communities that started after World War II. By the 1980s, the combination of federal neglect, the loss of the local tax base, the continuing constriction of municipal budgets, and outmigration of middle-class families had a deleterious effect on poor communities, particularly in the inner city (Halpern, 1995). The lack of resources to support community-based organizations (CBOs) and CBHOs, as well as other civic and social institutions, resulted in many ills, including entrenched racial and ethnic disparities in health that persist today. The trend of federal reductions in social and especially health spending continued through the 1990s and into the new century and is now aggressively implemented by the current administration, leaving the states with shrinking health care programs for the poor (Guiden, 2002).

Despite these difficulties, CBHOs continue to survive in the current precarious health care environment, although many concerns about them remain. Some observers fear that CBHOs will lose their character as vehicles of community involvement because their survival strategies make them a threat to civil society (Alexander, Nank, and Stivers, 1999). Others contend that CBHOs have become professionalized and that that very process has contributed to the demise of volunteerism in the United States (Beito, 1996). Equally pressing is the concern that the CBHOs most likely to succumb will be the ones that are most heavily dependent on government funding (Liebschutz, 1992).

The immediate response to the first concern is that CBHOs as a part of the health care system are operating in ways that are consistent with the times and the environment in which they function. Consequently, as a matter of survival, CBHOs must now adapt many practices, systems, and procedures from the for-profit world in order to provide evidence to public and private funders that they are accountable and efficient. An obvious response to the second concern is that political and economic conditions in the United States have conspired in such a way that even though we are all working harder, this does not always translate, particularly for the working poor, into doing better but instead into barely making it. As a result, more of the individuals coming off public assistance into low-paying jobs face the demand to work longer hours, which leaves them not only without time for volunteerism but worse, without time to supervise their children, and in the case of teenagers that spells disaster (Cornachio, 2003). Yet it is history that provides the clearest response to any concerns about the continued survival of CBHOs.

Conservative Views of Health Care for the Poor

Historically, the conservative position on health care and indeed most entitlement and benefit programs for citizens is that government should not be involved, and that thinking has held fast over the years. Current examples of conservative thinking on health care services reflect a variety of long-held beliefs (Hood, 2003):

- Americans must be offered ways to make their own health care arrangements without any government control.
- The new Child Health Insurance Program (CHIP) has added millions of nonpoor children to the rolls of Medicaid or Medicaid-like government programs.
- Americans want expanded personal choice and control over their health decisions.
- The preference of most Americans is for limited employer involvement in health care decision making.
- Since adding a prescription drug benefit to Medicare would be an unsustainable act of fiscal recklessness, the better approach is for seniors to pay for the increasing costs of drugs on their own.

- A viable solution to health coverage is the establishment of individually controlled health care savings accounts.

Two caveats follow from this conservative position. First is that any health care policies that result from this thinking will have the greatest negative impact on the poor, who are the clients of the majority of CBHOs, and therefore on the continued survival of CBHOs. The second is that the future of CBHOs calls for them to make very specific kinds of changes in response to clearly defined trends.

Of the CBHOs surveyed as part of the research conducted for this book, 77 percent came into existence since the 1970s, almost all (97 percent) serve low-income and uninsured patients, two-thirds of them (68 percent) serve large immigrant populations, and all nine of the CBHOs that were established after 1990 have budgets under $5 million. By comparison, the majority of organizations with budgets over $20 million (eight of eleven) were all established before 1980.

Admittedly, CBHO survival and growth are not easily accomplished and are dependent on a host of environmental factors. CBHOs struggle to survive in the face of massive changes in the social, cultural, political, economic, technological, and theoretical approaches that are giving shape to the health care industry of the future. Amid all of this change, CBHOs are caught between new demands for greater business efficiency and evidence-based improvements in health outcomes, on the one hand, and their ongoing commitment to community organizing, building, and empowerment, on the other. It is their ability to honor their commitments while making adaptations to changes that will shape the future of CBHOs.

CBHOs' Distinct Capacity for Change

CBHOs have consistently demonstrated a capacity to adapt to change. As a result of political decisions by the federal government in the 1960s to devolve the responsibility for health and social services to local government, new partnerships emerged between government and CBHOs. CBHOs rose to that challenge by growing both in number and in size and by serving as the training ground and employer of scores of community residents for whom employment in the private sector would have been difficult. Government cuts in the 1980s forced CBHOs to cut back programs and staff. CBHOs have responded to the frequent cutbacks since 2001 by implementing new measures.

As in the past, CBHOs confront these new challenges to their survival head on. We found evidence in our study, reported in Chapter Three, that they are working to buttress their organizations and ensure organizational survival. Some of the CBHOs we studied have instituted fee-for-service and where necessary have changed their mission statements. They are also working on maintaining relationships with elected officials, other organizations in the community, and the community at large as part of their advocacy efforts. Many of them are seeking and obtaining input and feedback from clients and using that input to inform ongoing staff training and grant writing as part of a community empowerment strategy. In addition, their preferred method of communicating with clients and the larger public is through the more personal format of community meetings.

These are all clear activities aimed at organizing, building, and empowering community. In the in-depth interview component of the research, CBHO administrators informed us that community organizing, building, and empowerment are critical to their ability to ensure organizational survival and growth. Without empowered communities and clients, it will be much more difficult for their organization to negotiate and develop innovative partnerships with other health care organizations and attract a diversified stream of public and private funding.

Therefore, the aim of this final chapter is to examine some of the current health challenges in the United States, to forecast some of the expected changes and trends that are projected to occur in health care delivery, and to share a vision for the future of CBHOs as a critical component of changes we envision in U.S. health care. To examine the shape of things to come, particularly of the role of CBHOs in the future of health care delivery in the United States, we draw on ideas from the international arena as well as ideas about community empowerment without which real partnerships, between multiple levels of a community, aimed at improving community health, cannot occur. Finally, this chapter is also intended to help redefine health-related research and health outcomes and to provide recommendations for the future of CBHOs that can contribute to the elimination of health disparities and to improved health for everyone.

Current Health Care Challenges

Over the course of the past century, the United States has faced and overcome numerous health challenges. Currently, the Centers for Disease Control and Prevention (CDC) lists ten public health goals for the twenty-first century (Koplan and Fleming, 2000, p. 284):

1. Institute a rational health care system.
2. Eliminate health disparities.
3. Focus on children's emotional and intellectual development.
4. Achieve a longer "healthspan."
5. Integrate physical activity and healthy eating into daily lives.
6. Clean up and protect the environment.
7. Prepare to respond to emerging infectious diseases.
8. Recognize and address the contributions of mental health to overall health and well-being.
9. Reduce the toll of violence in society.
10. Use new scientific knowledge and technological advances wisely.

The top two—to design a rational health care system and to eliminate health disparities—are closely linked, as they represent the major and most daunting challenge to government and health care systems in the United States. There is some consensus that the most rational system for health service delivery to the diverse populations in this country would be one in which everyone had access to some basic package of preventive and primary health care services (Rosenberg, 1997). Nevertheless, questions remain regarding how best to design a system that will be able to provide services in an efficient, cost-effective, culturally and linguistically appropriate manner that will serve to eliminate health disparities.

This challenge is complicated by biomedical knowledge, gained throughout the past century, of the etiology and progressive nature of health deterioration over time. Research related to this new knowledge has provided evidence that behavioral changes in areas such as nutrition, physical activity, and emotional and spiritual health are critical components of disease prevention and health improvement (Bayne Smith and others, 2004; Kaufman and Joseph-Fox, 1996). Therefore, if the United States is to achieve the CDC's top two goals, it must first address three critical health care challenges.

The first has to do with how best to influence and maintain changes in community health behavior, considering the extent to which health behavior and health practices are influenced by culture and community (Bayne Smith, 1999). The second has to do with redirecting a significant portion of health care resources, research agendas, mainstream institutional and organizational culture and behavior, and the overarching paradigms of the U.S. health care system toward achieving the first. The third challenge, also crucial to achieving the first, has to do with the willingness of the health care system to invest in community organizing, building, and empowerment as a precursor to the development of community-based partnerships, without which improvements in community health behaviors will not occur. The good news is that despite obstacles, multiple efforts to address all of these challenges are already under way.

For example, social and behavioral health problems such as domestic violence, gun violence, and teen births were considered thirty years ago to be private problems that were idiosyncratic of individuals and specific cultures. Today they are part of the public health agenda. Another example can be found in health-related preventive policies, such as smoke-free environments, enacted only in the past ten years to help curtail smoking among American adults. In addition, there are several interventions currently under way around the country consisting of policy and environmental changes designed to encourage healthy behaviors such as increased physical activity and healthy nutritional practices, decrease tobacco use, and reduce cardiovascular disease risk at the community and workplace level (Bayne Smith, 2002; Fisher and others, 1994; "Community Programs," 2000).

Further evidence of change is provided by one of the CBHOs in our study, reported in Chapter Three, that received initial startup funding from the National Institutes of Health (NIH) that was specifically earmarked to address the issue of homeless teens. The availability of NIH funds for service programs is evidence of change, as NIH has customarily focused on rigorous research involving double-blind clinical trials. A similar example can be found in the current Special Populations Grant from the Health Resources and Services

Administration (HRSA). Traditionally, HRSA, a service agency within the Department of Health and Human Services (DHHS), funds services. However, this most recent grant is focused primarily on research to test new models for providing peer support to HIV/AIDS patients in an effort to increase their adherence to treatment.

These examples make it clear that we have begun to expand not only the way we define health in the United States but also the ways in which we opt to address health issues.

Despite some movement in the right direction, it sometimes seems minimal and reluctant when compared to the huge pockets of resistance to change that continue to persist. This is most evident when efforts to address entrenched public health problems come up against well-organized opposition that hinders progress. For example, conservative resistance in the United States has managed to influence the development of public health policies that, unlike those in other developed nations, do not really help sexually active young people who for a variety of reasons opt to engage in risky behaviors. Current U.S. teen pregnancy prevention policies reflect our unwillingness to deal honestly and openly with issues such as teen sexuality. However, the situation is so serious and has so many implications for long-term poverty and mental and physical health problems for mothers and children that it cries out for better policy solutions at the national level.

Although community organizing, building, and empowerment work contributed to the decline in teen pregnancy rates during the 1990s, there are signs that the situation is changing. Based on emerging evidence that the decline is about to be reversed, the California Department of Finance predicts that the state's teen pregnancy rates will accelerate, leading to a 23 percent increase in teen births by 2008 (Delgado, 2003).

Outdated paradigms maintained by conservative forces that are bent on preserving the status quo have held back movement in other areas. For example, the vast majority of medical schools and other training programs for health professionals have been slow to devise more progressive curricula that will increase and improve interactions between providers and patients. This kind of training is vitally important, especially because so many medical schools and residency training programs are attached to large medical centers located in inner-city neighborhoods where care is likely to be delivered across lines of race, culture, and class. Equally in need of change are elitist attitudes and unwillingness at the academic, administrative, and managerial levels of the health care industry to recognize and value local knowledge in communities. These kinds of changes are crucial to changing the behavior of health professionals, which will lead to reciprocal behavior changes on the part of patients.

Recognition of the ability of CBHOs to provide health education and health promotion and of the safety net role that they play for groups both rural and urban with Medicaid or no insurance is growing (Irigoyen and Findley, 1998; Forrest and Whelan, 2000). But some CBHOs and other nonprofits do not have the necessary structures and systems (management information systems, accounting, human resources) or the required level of organizational capacity (board of directors, mission statement, strategic plans) for long-term effectiveness (Fredericksen and London, 2000). Nevertheless, there is little evidence that funders have made any commitment to funding CBHOs and other nonprofits to build their organizational structures and overall capacity.

Even public health professionals who are becoming more accepting of community-based approaches to public health admit that they are hampered by the health systems they work for, which have different structures than those that exist in the community, and by their limited understanding of how to approach community and their misguided focus on assets rather than on needs and deficiencies (McKnight, 2000). Other health professionals have also become more accepting of the need for development of partnerships with CBHOs, especially those that provide health education services. However, they do not always understand that partnerships with these types of CBHOs can lead to effective teaching and learning opportunities for faculty, staff, and the community at large (Bruce, McKane, and Brock, 2000).

Recently, the American Public Health Association (APHA) and the W. K. Kellogg Foundation collaborated to share results of the Kellogg program on community-based public health. This program was designed to create partnerships between community-based organizations and public health departments as well as schools of public health, medicine, nursing, and social work. The most impressive result of this initiative was the number of courses and opportunities provided to students, faculty, and staff at the involved schools to learn more about community (Bruce, McKane, and Brock, 2000). The Kellogg initiative is part of a new trend indicating a growing awareness of the need to provide health professionals with a more comprehensive education that is mindful of the wider range of community needs and the importance of working in partnership with communities to address health needs (O'Neil, 1993; Morrison and others, 1997).

The progressive trends we have mentioned are indeed encouraging. However, it must be noted that at the root of persistent health disparities is the entrenched poverty in which so many communities in the United States and indeed around the world find themselves mired. For these people, very little, if anything, is being done to address that more recalcitrant problem. Income disparities between those on top and those on the bottom are such that the number of people living in extreme circumstances (less than $6,750 per year for a family of three) increased from 13.9 million in 1995 to 14.6 million in 1997 (Gergen, 1999, p. 64).

This trend of increasing poverty and how that is connected to poor health is supported by recent census data released by the Center on Budget and Policy Priorities (CBPP) in 2004, which show that the number and percentage of Americans living below the poverty line increased every year between 2000 and 2003 and that the number and percentage of people without health insurance also climbed in each of those years. This increase in poverty was the largest since record keeping began in 1987. Since 2000, the year before unemployment began to rise, the number of people in poverty has risen by 4.3 million while median income has fallen by $1,535, after adjustment for inflation, and the number of people with no health insurance has increased by 5.2 million (Center on Budget and Policy Priorities, 2004).

Further, as of October 2003, there were 2.1 million people looking for but unable to find full-time work, while another 5 million people were working part-time because they too could not find full-time employment (Leonhardt, 2003). The connection between persistent poverty and persistent poor health has been made repeatedly in this book. Suffice it to say that without a commitment to simultaneously tackling these twin evils, the advances being made in only one of them, improvements in health care for poor communities, is unlikely to have the desired effects. In the United States and around the world, efforts to remove health disparities must now be backed up by resources and wider political and economic changes that directly address endemic poverty (Gordon, 1995).

Forecasting Changes in U.S. Health Care: The Viability of CBHOs

Given the various trends just discussed and the relentless pace at which new trends evolve and change occurs, CBHOs are understandably concerned about what to expect in the future. Yet the need to plan makes it is necessary to examine current trends in terms of their projected influence on health care delivery in the future. At recent health care forums and policy discussions, we asked academics, funders of CBHOs, foundation staff, government policy wonks, and staff and board members of various health care organizations to forecast trends they believe will affect CBHOs in the next ten to twelve years. Our synthesis of their responses is presented next.

Changing Trends

The future is certain to hold more of the sociocultural, political, and economic changes that began with the liberal federal health initiatives of the 1960s and the reliance on technology for health service delivery and health planning that began in the 1970s and 1980s. McBride (1994) chronicled these changes, pointing presciently to the twin problems we see today—lack of access for increasing numbers of the poor and uninsured and persistent health disparities in specific diseases that had become evident by the mid-1980s.

This trend has indeed continued, albeit with new twists. The economic and social issues of health care access and health disparities have been exacerbated by political action in the form of immigration reforms, welfare reform, and health care reform. Since 2001, the Bush administration has increased the customary fiscal troubles of most cities and thrown some of them into budgetary crisis through ever more aggressive efforts to curtail Medicaid and education spending.

The recent legislative reforms reflect conservative political agendas that are fueled by racism and xenophobia. Legislation is essentially strategic behavior by individuals who refuse to acknowledge that nearly every resident of the United States today got here as a result of immigration. But more important than immigrant status is the question of time of arrival. Those who got here first were in the position of being able to seize more, and by virtue of that early position, they were also able to relegate everyone else—those who were here initially but were vanquished and all those who came after—to secondary or even lesser status by designing and dominating the political and economic framework through which policy decisions are made, implemented, and enforced.

Essentially, then, the legislative reforms of the 1970s, 1980s, and 1990s provide evidence of a conservative trend involving the cultural, political, and economic reassertion, following their brief moratorium in the 1960s, of those who got here first. Conservatism as a trend is critically important for the following reason: for the foreseeable future, trends involving government decreases in social spending, accompanied by ongoing devolution of responsibility for social problems to the states, is expected to continue, irrespective of whether elections are won by Democrats or Republicans.

The confluence of these social, political, and economic trends has already triggered awareness in some poor communities and outright movement in others. For example, senior staff of community-based agencies around the nation that are involved in the Kellogg Foundation's Families and Neighborhoods initiative participated in a research project in which they offered specific recommendations on how Kellogg might help its grantees address community needs in the aftermath of welfare reform (Withorn and Jons, 1999). Participant recommendations included the need for recognition and meaningful inclusion of community voices in policy discussions and decisions, greater levels of assistance in meeting constituency needs and new policy mandates, understanding and responding to increased poverty among working poor, assistance in serving people who have lost income and are unable to find work, assistance in keeping connected to other CBOs and avoiding isolation, and more focused funding that will support community outreach, organizing building, leadership development, and ultimately empowerment.

On the rare occasions when they are asked, poor communities, especially poor communities of color, are very clear on what they need: jobs, housing, child care, economic revival of the inner cities, better health care and welfare systems, fair immigration laws, and good-quality education (Rivera and Erlich, 1998). For example, a recent study commissioned by a group of foundations in the nation's capital used an in-depth interview format to investigate the need for a consumer health advocacy group and to obtain input from community residents on how best to design such an entity. Participants included consumers, community activists and residents, staff of CBOs involved in advocacy, staff of foundations, and consultants to foundations in the District of Columbia. They unanimously agreed on the need for a consumer health advocacy organization (Bayne Smith and Perot, 2003). Many of the interviewees have a history of continuous organizing involvement in the district. All of them were passionately clear in their recommendations to foundations. They suggested that the proposed consumer advocacy organization should be community-based, supported by participating foundations to engage in community organizing, building, and empowerment at various levels of community, and that these activities must include training, leadership development, and skills development that can lead to employment in the private sector.

New social movements are also under way. In a recent interview, the executive director of a clinic serving Hispanic immigrant populations indicated that although the clinic provides health services, much of what he does is also about community organizing and building. He explained that the clinic is committed to the continuous education of its immigrant clients about health promotion practices and behaviors as well as providing information about their right to health care. He also advises them of their civil rights, though immigrants, as residents and citizens of the United States. He did issue a caveat that organizing with new immigrants from Latin America is different. One has to be mindful of their history and of cultural norms that do not encourage any behavior that appears to challenge authority. He also noted that they tend to feel fearful because they are monolingual in Spanish, which prevents them from clearly expressing their input. If undocumented, they prefer to remain invisible.

Probably the most encouraging trend is that immigrants' rights groups are organizing around the country and in different parts of the world to make their needs known. Those needs often include equal pay for equal work as well as the need for health care services. Most recently, approximately 100,000 immigrants came together in New York City from all over the United States, Mexico, China, Haiti, and other countries to stage a rally in Flushing Meadow Park, Queens. Their goal was to persuade policymakers in Congress to grant legal status to more than 8 million immigrants, to issue more family unification visas, to provide increased work protections for immigrants who are exploited by employers, and to end the civil liberties violations against them that have been occurring since September 11, 2001. The most interesting component of this national and international campaign for immigrants' rights is their sources of support, which includes labor unions and the Catholic church (Greenhouse, 2003).

Based on this discussion of social and cultural trends and changes in U.S. health care, the viability of CBHOs as entities that provide services primarily to poor, uninsured, and immigrant populations can be safely forecast. To begin with, health care advocates succeeded in pressuring government to delink Medicaid from welfare assistance such as Temporary Assistance to Needy Families. Many states had reasonably projected that thanks to the ending of welfare, they would be able to handle the increased costs of Medicaid. Indeed, some of states increased eligibility for Medicaid to 200 percent of the poverty level, and in a small number of states, eligibility is as high as 300 percent. The current benefit of increased coverage is, of course, that more whole families among the working poor are covered: mothers are covered through Medicaid, and CHIP covers children under eighteen years of age in most states and under nineteen in a few. For the moment, this trend seems secure in that it has spread to all of the states. However, advocates must keep the pressure on because additional federal cuts in Medicaid seem certain. Needless to say, further economic erosion will force states to address budget deficits, and one of the most likely areas state and local policymakers will sacrifice in an effort to achieve a balanced budget will almost certainly be health care services.

Should the current trend persist, however, Medicaid enrollments will increase but states will continue to insist that Medicaid clients receive their health care services through Medicaid Managed Care (MMC) companies or some form of capitated, market-controlled financing system. This brings us to a new trend, which is the development of partnerships and business agreements between CBHOs, managed care entities, and other partners. These partnerships are expected to be of two kinds: CBHO–Medicaid Managed Care partnerships and CHC–managed care partnerships.

CBHO-MMC Partnerships

The first and easier type of partnership to configure will be between CBHOs that do not deliver clinical care and MMC companies as private enterprises. The fact that they will come together not as competitors but as collaborators will serve to facilitate these kinds of partnerships. Therefore, it seems safe to predict that CBHOs that provide preventive services such as health-related outreach, education, enrollment, peer support services, social and support services, and case management will begin to forge partnerships or increase the terms of existing agreements with MMC entities and other partners as well.

These partnerships and business arrangements are predicted to increase because as strategic collaborations between nonprofits and businesses, they make good business sense. They can be structured to start out at any point along a continuum that moves from a onetime philanthropic interaction to a more transactional relationship that is analogous to a buyer-seller relationship on to an integrated relationship that is personal and collective (Austin, 2000). The goal for CBHOs as we move forward must be to seek transactional and integrated relationships with MMC companies as equal partners.

These relationships are predicted to be successful because both CBHOs and MMC companies need these types of partnerships at this time in their development, given the current aggressive health care financing climate. CBHOs have valuable services that MMC companies will be more willing to purchase as they face increasing pressure in the future to improve health outcomes for their enrollees. MMC entities are very aware that health outcomes improve through the practice of preventive care, but they offer primary care services. Further, most, if not all, MMC organizations are not community-based and tend to have minimal information about the history and culture of the community in which they are established and for whom they have accepted the responsibility to serve (Schacht, 1998).

As a result, partnerships between CBHOs and the MMC companies are mutually beneficial. MMC organizations can benefit greatly from the help of community insiders such as CBHOs to assist them penetrate communities that are culturally different and by connecting those clients in designated target populations to MMC programs. CBHOs will benefit from partnerships with MMC companies in which they are able to contribute to improving the health of their community and at the same time preserve their organizations.

CHC-MC Partnerships

The other type of partnership is very different. It involves federally funded community health centers, which are a type of CBHO that delivers clinical care. CHCs have had some struggles with coming under the managed care umbrella as the nation moved from fee-for-service to managed care (MC). In making the transition to managed care, CHCs had to rely on their advocacy networks to enter into the fray at national, state, and local policy levels and bargaining tables to protect local community clinics, clinical providers, staff, and the services that the vulnerable and underserved populations they take care of depend on. In the process of that struggle, CHCs have continued to work collaboratively with various levels of government and through their networks to share resources and information on policy developments in health reform (Schauffler and Wolin, 1996). To date, CHCs have escaped budget cuts and continue to survive and grow.

As CBHOs develop partnerships with MMC organizations or other partners at national, state, and local levels and as they seek help from funders to continue meeting the needs of their constituents and to develop or increase their advocacy functions, the issue of capacity will have to be dealt with (Fredericksen and London, 2000). Some local funders have begun to talk about the importance of providing funding not only for organizational capacity building but also for community organizing, building, and empowerment. It can be predicted that as we go forward, others, including some of the national foundations, will also come to see the need to bolster the operations of CBHOs and to assist local efforts to carefully plan and strategize around community empowerment for the poor. Without strong structures, internal operating capacity, and an empowered constituency, CBHOs will fail.

Shifting Theoretical Perspectives

For more than a century, medicine and indeed the entire health care industry enjoyed what is probably the highest professional status in U.S. society. The expertise power of physicians went unquestioned for decades, and the hegemony of the medical model was completely autonomous in its ability to diagnose, prescribe treatment, and insist on medical compliance. But that has begun to change. And one area where change is clearly evident is in the relationship of women to the health care system.

Despite the seemingly limitless power of doctors and the health industry, women struggled since the mid-1800s against the medicalization of naturally occurring phenomena connected to their bodies at different points in the life cycle (Ehrenreich and English, 1973). The intense level of organization, civic participation, and community empowerment of the 1960s reenergized the women's health movement, and with it came many challenges to medical authority. What followed was an increasing use of complementary and alternative medicine, from acupuncture to midwives. Indeed, the entire field of alternative medicine is another area of radical change.

Today, the National Center for Complementary and Alternative Medicine (NCCAM) is one of the twenty-seven institutes and centers that make up the National Institutes of Health. NCCAM was established by Congress in 1998. It conducts research, research training and career development, outreach, and integration of scientifically proven complementary and alternative medicine (CAM) practices into conventional medicine. It also supports programs to develop models for incorporating CAM into the curriculum of medical, dental, and nursing schools. Appropriations for each fiscal year from Congress can be viewed on the Web at http://nccam. nih.gov/about/appropriations.

Since the 1960s, complementary and alternative medicine, or healing, has come to refer much less to issues of health care and much more so to a focus on prevention and management of health conditions. This new thinking initiated a slow but increasing shift away from the medical model to a broader definition of health and a nascent but growing understanding of the complexity of multi-level ecological systems that affect community health. From the perspective of ecological theory, health care must take now on a more comprehensive systems approach that examines and treats the whole person, and the CAM approach fits well with ecological theory. It can be expected, then, that CAM assessments of individual patients will include queries regarding community health and environment quality, lifestyle and health behavior practices, spiritual and emotional assets or deficits, quality of nutritional practices, levels of physical activity, genetic structure, and the many other components that make for healthy living.

While the CAM changes represent one aspect of the broader context of changes in health care, it now appears that the general orientation toward disease, treatment, and cures has begun to shift toward health promotion, prevention, and wellness. Admittedly, this shift has been influenced by new thinking that is closely linked to the CAM approach. Yet there are limits to the CAM approach. It is not designed to address any of the fundamental contributing sources of poor health, such as poverty, environmental and social justice, or the kinds of difficulties experienced by providers in treating those that are not of the same class, race, and gender of the provider.

Amid the various changing perceptions and orientations, CBHOs stand out as the most viable component of the health care system for delivery of preventive, wellness, and advocacy services for racial and ethnic minorities, immigrants, and women of all ages. CBHOs are poised to take on more of that role as we go forward. As community-based entities, CBHOs are fully aware of the CAM health practices of their community and in some instances are even part of them. In addition, CBHOs as entities embedded in a community, are in the enviable position of being trusted with information regarding client use of culturally sanctioned healers and age-old health practices, which is information that is not likely to be shared with mainstream providers (Randall-David, 1989). Moreover, as community residents, most CBHO staff and some providers are also affected by the complex issues involved with health and health care for residents, including levels of poverty, violence, and other social and environmental dangers. All of these factors make CBHOs more attuned to the multiple issues affecting the whole of people's lives.

Finally, and most significant, CBHOs enjoy the respect and trust of their clients. They are known in their communities and are counted on to deliver a wide array of outreach, education, peer support, and case management services, all of which double as hands-on methods for engaging people, providing them with a model to emulate, and helping them practice preventive behaviors. It can safely be predicted that CBHOs are well suited for a growing role in the prevention and wellness model of care that is expected to dominate in the future.

New Research and Scientific Approaches

Probably the most entrenched part of the U.S. health system and therefore the most resistant to change is the scientific research community. Many of the research procedures used by health care program planners and pharmaceutical companies have been around for half a century and were established to preserve the purity of every aspect of a research project, from the sampling of participants to the presentation of results. The goal of scientific research methodologies such as double-blind clinical trials is to keep the research free, at every step of the way, from contamination by either the investigator or the subjects. These research methods and procedures are effectively designed for use in clinical trials to test whether new pharmaceutical products or treatments are suitable for widespread use. Variations are also used for evaluation research testing whether an intervention is effective and therefore worthy of replication. These research methods are quite suitable for the testing of new products, but there is some concern about their usefulness for evaluating an intervention to determine effectiveness or replication merit.

Other criticisms apply to who customarily does the research and the roles to which subjects are traditionally relegated in research projects. For example, the research methods used in clinical trials have long been criticized as being too costly and inadequate in that the most valuable information they provide is about averages. As a result of our new understanding of the sequence of the human genome, these research methods are also being criticized as outmoded because the data obtained are not specific enough to properly treat people who depart from the average. In contrast, genomics data will allow physicians in the future to tailor treatment to individual biological makeup.

Another criticism of older research practices surrounds the use of research subjects who participate only at the point of data gathering, after which they are ignored. The new research framework calls for the involvement of multiple levels of community, including residents, health workers, policymakers, and other stakeholders in the various areas and stages of research. This process is thought to provide greater accuracy in research. The involvement of multiple levels of community provides an opportunity to test in one community segment the accuracy of responses from another.

For example, participatory baseline research was conducted across the five sites of the Plain Talk/Hablando Claro program, a community-based initiative of the Annie E. Casey Foundation designed to reduce teen pregnancies, STDs, and HIV/AIDS that is now in the dissemination and replication phase. At baseline, parents reported that they talked to their teenagers about sex and sexuality. Their teenagers, surveyed separately from parents, reported that parents did not give them accurate, adequate, or sufficient information. Surveyors, hired from within the community, were able to return to the community to share information with adults about problems *the community's own* children had expressed. This involvement of multiple levels of a community not only increased the accuracy of responses but also was instrumental in gaining acceptance from community adults. More important in terms of outcomes, participatory research methods helped improve and increase communication between adults and sexually active youth and ultimately helped reduce risky behavior among youth and even some adults in those communities (Grossman, Walker, Kotloff, and Pepper, 2001).

The level and pace of community change accomplished in each of the Plain Talk/Hablando Claro communities was directly commensurate with the extent to which the CBO or CBHO in which the program was housed was embedded in its community. CBO and CBHO connectedness to community was also crucial in terms of facilitating the participatory research conducted for this program. Participatory research and evaluation are now internationally recognized as a more effective research approach for assessing quality and providing evidence of effectiveness of interventions (Speak, 2000). Participatory research methods are projected to increase in the future. CBHOs, particularly those that engage in community organizing, building, and empowerment, are well positioned to serve as base organizations for conducting participatory research at multiple levels in a community. Even more important, CBHOs need to develop skills and expertise in data and problem analysis, as without it they are hard pressed to definitively adopt or defend an economic, political, social justice, legal, or principled position on an issue.

Envisioning Healthy Communities

Over the past few decades has come a slow recognition that reliance on diagnosis and treatment of disease is insufficient. We are becoming aware that biological technologies alone will not eliminate chronic disease and that these are more likely to continue increasing the cost of care. Therefore, projections are for a shift toward prevention and health promotion. This process is also about broadening the definition of health beyond a singular focus on individual responsibility for good health. Understanding is now emerging that good health is a community phenomenon. As a result, prevention and health promotion must target not only the whole person but also, to the extent possible, the community conditions and context in which the person lives.

The work of creating healthy communities is essentially the work of community organizing, building, and empowerment that builds social capital and social cohesion and leads to group empowerment and the confidence to create a vision of what people want their future health status, life, and community to be. A good example of local efforts to create healthy communities can be found in the ongoing organizing work being done with Native Americans around self-determination, self-governance, and positive cultural identification. In a study of the Salt Lake Native American community, a vision for future development was collectively created, clarified, re-created, and eventually integrated into the hearts and minds of the community (Edwards and Egbert-Edwards, 1998). That trend of rebuilding, empowering, and creating a future vision for the Native American community is quite active in the United States today.

The work of envisioning a healthy community is also being accomplished beyond the local level. A national survey conducted in 1985 to determine the health status of minorities revealed serious heath disparities (Heckler, 1985). The report of that survey was subsequently used by the Public Health Service and other government agencies at the federal level to set up the national program known initially as the Healthy People Consortium. That program laid the groundwork for future trends in monitoring and establishing targets and in subsequently moving the nation toward improved health that started with the work of the Healthy People 2000 guidelines and now continues with Healthy People 2010.

In the CBHO study reported in Chapter Three, many participants indicated that they engaged in advocacy and community empowerment. The very process of establishing CBHOs requires that a community, or at least its leaders, create a vision of the kind of future health status and health services the community wants and deserves. CBHOs play a critical role in creating a future vision of health for a community because so much of the work that is done, in addition to providing services, is about organizing the community around a future vision and involving residents and other stakeholders in bringing that vision to fruition. Many of the individuals interviewed in our CBHO study told stories of additional work that had to be put into their local health system to make them more receptive to the visions communities had for improving their future health conditions. It was clear that in the process of establishing a CBHO, communities were brought together around a variety of issues, including vision, mission, scope of services to be offered, partnerships, and funding.

Transformations in U.S. Health Systems

The foregoing discussion clearly indicates that the U.S. health care system is projected to adapt a preventive health delivery model. Also clear but probably harder to achieve because of long-standing and systemic investments is that we will need new theoretical paradigms. For example, there is increasing agreement that preventive services and preventive strategies that include behavior change are the way of the future. However, there is less consensus that prevention policies and programs will not be adequately supported by the old mechanistic paradigm of the biomedical model and that it is time to embrace a more comprehensive perspective such as the biopsychosocial model or an approach that rests on ecological or systems theory. Either of these theoretical approaches offers a more useful framework for developing a new health and sociomedical model that will be able to address the comprehensive needs of the whole person living in a community.

Probably the most difficult area of prevention that the new system will have to address is behavior change, on the part of not just patients but providers as well. Although it can be expected that there will be challenges in any effort to change behavior, we now have ample behavior change models for individuals, specific populations, and communities (Proschaska and Velicer, 1997; Kegeles, Hays, and Coates, 1996; Kelly, Saint Lawrence, and Stevenson, 1992).

Given that physician behavior change efforts remain an underdeveloped area, a new trend that is likely to occur, particularly in managed care settings, will be physician participation in behavioral change programs. Compliance will be obtained by linking physician program participation to outcome measures because pressure is projected to increase on managed care companies as demands mount for greater accountability and improved health outcomes for the clients they serve. Without this kind of pressure, provider behavior is not expected to change very much. The training required to assist providers with learning to handle their own behavioral issues in relating to patients should be part of mandated medical school curricula. However, it can be expected that the institutions that train our health professionals, especially the medical schools, will be the very last arenas in which change will occur.

Transformation of the U.S. health system is also expected to occur in mental health service delivery, particularly for the poor, communities of color, and immigrant populations. The level of disinvestment in poor communities, especially communities of color, creates intolerable conditions that are conducive to mental health problems. Therefore, future providers of mental health services to communities of color will have to be mindful of the level of deterioration and its impact on community residents, on the one hand, as well as the stigma attached to these services by people of color, on the other (Clark-Amankwaa, 2003). It will also be important to recognize as we go forward that mental health services provided from a predominantly European mind-set is less helpful than services delivered in settings and using approaches that are more culturally sensitive.

The projected changes that are expected to occur in the U.S. health system of the future may appear radical to some. However, health systems, like all other systems in the modern age, are in a state of continuous flux. Think back to December 10, 1948, when the General Assembly of the United Nations proclaimed the Universal Declaration of Human Rights. Article 25 of that declaration seemed wildly utopian at the time: "Everyone has the right to a standard of living adequate for the health and well-being of himself and of his family, including food, clothing, housing and medical care and necessary social services, and the right to security in the event of unemployment, sickness, disability, widowhood, old or other lack of livelihood in circumstances beyond his control." Yet since then, Article 25 has been used around the world as the basis for advocacy, community empowerment, and creating a vision for healthy communities.

International Efforts

After adoption of the Universal Declaration of Human Rights, the World Health Organization (WHO) and the United Nations, as international organizations, went on to develop programs aimed at engendering healthy communities. These programs were premised on an assumed basic human right to health care, without which it is not possible to strive for a good and fulfilled life. The World Health Assembly set the goal of "Health for All by the Year 2000." By 1991, despite concerns regarding the extent to which Health for All by 2000 was being derailed by politics, elite group issues, and lack of community participation, the feeling was that it was still attainable (Green, 1991).

Since then, the WHO's 2002 *World Health Report* (Brundtland, 2002) indicated, the greatest burden of health risks has continued to be borne by the poorest peoples of the world (in Nigeria, Guatemala, Native America, Ethiopia, Zimbabwe, Colombia, Haiti, Bangladesh, the Philippines, and Puerto Rico). The report also indicated that the burden is greatest for the most disadvantaged members in every society and that the vast majority of threats to health are commonly found in communities where there are concentrations of people with little education and low-income occupations. The report cautions that if we are to create healthy communities, the negative health conditions of poor people must be addressed on three fronts: governments will have to take on more responsibility for health risk reduction, work has to be done with individuals and communities to improve their health, and efforts must be made with the providers who serve them to help them do so in more effective ways.

The call for a balanced approach among government, individuals and community, and providers and service organizations has been most efficiently responded to by nongovernmental organizations (NGOs) rather than local governments. In poor countries all over the world, NGOs have helped the poor organize, develop joint income-generating activities, and become empowered. Working with poor people in developing countries to implement and sustain income-producing or time-saving activities is both labor-intensive and costly. Therefore, NGOs operate in poor countries primarily on external funding. NGOs are able to provide well-trained field staff who commit to spending years working closely with the poor, becoming immersed in local knowledge, and ultimately gaining trust (Galjart, 1995). As a result of their commitment to joint planning with the poor and their long-term commitment to the projects they undertake, NGOs have acquired full cooperation from such funding streams as the World Bank and the Inter-American Foundation (IAF), which is an independent foreign assistance agency of the U.S. government.

Mayo and Craig (1995) describe four broad categories of NGOs, also known as private voluntary organizations, in the United States: international NGOs that are based in the West, government-sponsored agencies that support work in different parts of the world, voluntary organizations that provide contractual public services internationally, and grassroots development organizations. These four kinds of NGOs provide a variety of services that include relief, welfare, advocacy, networking, and campaigning. In some instances, combinations of these services are provided as part of a strategy to increase community participation and empowerment.

Two particular categories of NGOs and the trends they represent are worthy of mention: grassroots support organizations (GSOs) and membership support organizations (MSOs). The major distinction between GSOs and MSOs is that there is no direct accountability between a GSO (an outside group) and the people they support, whereas MSOs (an insider group) are directly accountable to their members. GSOs and MSOs are distinguished from NGOs primarily by the fact that the former operate within the country on which they focus, while most other NGOs are international, providing services in a developing country but based in a developed country (Carroll, 1992).

NGOs have been around for half a century, and they have come to be viewed as favorable conduits for international giving, especially from the IAF. The IAF provides grants to NGOs and CBOs in Latin America and the Caribbean to support innovative, sustainable, and participatory self-help programs. The IAF funds partnerships between grassroots organizations, nonprofits, businesses, and local governments throughout the Americas. One IAF-funded NGO doing grassroots health improvement work in a rural area of Panama in the early 1980s demonstrated that it was possible to shift the attention of health systems within a country from curative to preventive health services (Carroll, 1992). This was accomplished essentially by working to organize and build the level of participation of rural Panamanian communities in the design, development, and implementation of their vision of better community health.

NGOs are the international counterparts of U.S.-based CBOs and CBHOs. The similarity between these organizations lies in their common work of providing services and support to poor local communities, sometimes linking their clients to other local groups, and in most instances organizing the poor to become empowered. These organizations do not replace government because they cannot make policy. What they can do is help poor people take incremental steps toward empowerment, improved health, and in some cases small-scale economic development (Galjart, 1995).

Discussing possible projections for the future of health service delivery globally, Jong-Wook Lee (2003), the director general of the World Health Organization, issued a call for cooperation among all nations. He asked that science, moral vision, and political courage be applied to the task, which has the following goals:

- Recognizing health as an absolute human need and society's obligation to provide for all its members as best it can
- Supporting countries in building health systems that can provide reliable basic care that meets the needs of all their residents
- Developing a focus on primary care, with global targets in nutrition, maternal and child health, and access to essential medicines
- Control of communicable diseases, especially HIV/AIDS, with the specific goal of getting a minimum of three million people

in developing countries on antiretroviral combination therapy by the end of 2005.

Community Empowerment

Community empowerment is a collective effort that is crucial to achieving health goals and healthy communities in general. The essential principle of community empowerment rests on the use of organizing strategies to get communities to take responsibility for their health. Community organizing around empowerment leads to participation and involvement as well as exploration and understanding of the underlying issues associated with poor health. Not only do these underlying issues serve an organizing function, but focusing on them can have the greatest impact on improving health.

Community Empowerment: The Freire Method

The work of Paulo Freire with the poor in Latin America provides a useful model that may help organizing efforts with diverse groups in the United States. Freire took a two-pronged approach: a teaching style based on adult education methodologies combined with an organizing strategy designed to increase social and political awareness. The end goal of the Freirean model is the development of critical consciousness, increased community participation, and community empowerment.

The emphasis on developing critical consciousness in the Freire method is especially useful for working across cultures and other divisions. Community participation and empowerment involve focusing initially on the whole person. Thus the development of critical consciousness starts by focusing on the individual, moves on to small groups, and eventually encompasses the whole community. This is important because the great diversity of people in the United States who are poor, uninsured, immigrants, members of racial and ethnic minorities, or otherwise disfranchised impairs their ability to join forces. Factors that keep them apart include race, language, educational and income levels, religion, and allegiances to countries of origin.

In addition to the many ways in which marginalized groups divide themselves, they are further encouraged to maintain their divisions in a variety of ways. For example, in U.S. society, teachers and other professionals, and especially the media, exacerbate group divisions by portraying one group as the model minority, insisting that some groups are better suited to certain occupations and professions than others, and implying that certain groups commit much or all of the crime. As a result, marginalized peoples remain focused on what divides them, thereby failing to address their common issues of political, social, and economic powerlessness. Nor do they develop strategies on how to increase their political power or to leverage the power of their numbers to influence the political system. Consequently, goals for organizing and empowering groups of diverse people have not been easy to develop.

Working with diverse groups calls for partnerships that are committed to a process of ongoing learning and teaching, understanding, and constructive conflict resolution as the partners build, organize, and further develop community. The concepts of learning from and teaching each other are an outgrowth of Freire's work. In *Pedagogy of the Oppressed,* Freire (1990) argues that true partnership is a mutual process without which true development cannot occur.

CBHOs have long understood and applied variations of the Freire methodology. Many of those CBHOs that participated in the study reported in Chapter Three use a multipronged approach to service delivery in which they provide health and health-related services, as well as community organizing, building, and empowerment activities that include health education related to the services they provide, dissemination of communitywide prevention and health promotion messages, and information through flyers, brochures, community meetings, and a variety of other media. Some of the CBHOs in the study were also engaged in advocacy activities and efforts to organize their clients.

However, CBHOs can enhance their use of the Freire method. They must now jointly develop with the community well-crafted plans that will incorporate, shape, and guide more accurate replications of the twin components of the Freire model: adult education about the various health issues affecting their distinct community and an organizing effort designed to raise social and political consciousness among individuals and eventually the community as a whole.

Community Empowerment: The CBHO Intervention Model

In addition to a more careful replication of the Freire method, CBHOs must now rigorously evaluate how they are using this model and organize to institutionalize the model throughout the health care system serving their community. Finally, CBHOs would be wise to seek support for comprehensive programs that address the full spectrum of individual lives and community need for services, education, and community empowerment and participation. The difficulty here is that whereas community building through CBHOs is influenced by a host of factors related to the community in question, as well as the characteristics of both the community-building process and the organizers themselves (Mattessich and Monsey, 2001), health care funding in the United States, both public and private, is provided in isolated "silos" for specific health issues such as HIV/AIDS, diabetes, or asthma.

A model for building vibrant communities that closely resembles the CBHO intervention model of community building and empowerment was presented at a January 2003 meeting for Caribbean elected and appointed officials by Jerry Kolo of the Florida Atlantic University Center for Urban Redevelopment and Empowerment. In this model, different stakeholder sectors have different basic roles. The model also includes four sets of goals—physical, psychosocial, economic, and political—and accomplishing each set requires organizing with different sectors of the community.

Physical Goals

Physical goals encompass basic human needs such as food, shelter, housing, safety and security, health care, and education. Accomplishing these goals requires partnership among the communities, CBOs and CBHOs, the public, private, and philanthropic sectors, and legislators, all working to ensure that policies are enacted and programs are available for affordable housing, safety net programs, and health and social services.

It is important to expand here on the subject of education, as ideas about education differ. Education is considered one of the most important institutions of any society. In the United States, all groups have traveled through the education system, but outcomes have been very different for different groups. Part of the reason, as noted in Chapter Two, is that the highest quality of education in the nation has always been available only in the most prestigious schools. Thus where one obtains an education has the ability to empower or oppress.

Therefore, in the context of community empowerment, especially among people who have been miseducated, the need is for an educational approach that is very different from traditional practices in which a teacher or expert lectures and instructs less knowledgeable students. On the contrary, education for community empowerment and health improvement requires the willingness on the part of both teacher and student to learn from and teach each other.

Psychosocial Goals

Self-awareness and cultural awareness, acculturation and social integration, and civic participation are among the psychosocial goals that contribute to community empowerment. Community is built slowly, one resident at a time. As self-awareness and cultural awareness are awakened, people gain greater understanding of social, political, civic, and economic realities. They are then able to recognize the value of joining with other like-minded residents to question existing conditions such as the lack of access to health care for those who are poor, immigrant, and uninsured, to seek answers, and to work toward social change.

Economic Goals

The economy has large and profound effects not only on the quality of people's lives but also on the political actions of government, thereby creating an intricate relationship between the political system and the economic system (Cohen, 2000). It can be assumed that everyone aspires to similar economic goals. However, the political and government interrelationships with the economy make the achievement of economic goals vastly different from one community to another. The achievement of economic goals in any given community requires opportunities for high-quality education, gainful employment, creating wealth, gaining technological skills, and bolstering self-sufficiency. For residents of poor communities where there are negligible economic investments and opportunities, the emphasis must be on developing organized, targeted interventions to educate residents about the relationship between economic empowerment and improved health.

Political Goals

Understanding and using the political process and understanding one's human and health care rights and civil liberties are some key indicators of community empowerment. Present difficulties in cross-group organizing notwithstanding, if health care is to become available to all in the United States, it will happen as a result of an organizing groundswell. Organized power is required to bring the necessary pressure to bear on elected officials, as it is unlikely that they will muster the political will and courage to do so without a demand. However, organizing around the goal of health care for all cannot be effective if confined to any one group or population segment. Indeed, the future of community organizing and empowerment in the United States, whether it be for health or for any other universally beneficial issue, will have to be done across lines of race, class, religion, and all the other areas of diversity. Cross-group organizing represents the new frontier in the field, and it calls for different models than the ones that have been used in the past.

These goals are accomplished through community empowerment, specifically political empowerment, which has been shown to have an impact on health status (LaViest, 1992). Immigrants were at one time reluctant to become U.S. citizens based on the view that this represented a disloyal act against their country of origin. Nevertheless, many immigrants opted to become citizens much more out of a desire to increase their opportunity to sponsor relatives and reunite families than any desire to vote. However, as a result of immigration reforms and the loss of benefits, many immigrants obtained a crash course in the U.S. political process and what citizenship means in terms of a community's capacity to advocate for its fair share. The latest trend in immigrant communities is to acquire U.S. citizenship as soon as one is eligible to do so.

The importance of political goals and political participation must also be understood in terms of what is happening in the broader arena, particularly as it relates to health and health care. With the advent of jet travel, the world has become one large global community. This is a significant development with literally far-flung implications for disease transmission. From a health perspective, national or political borders are nonexistent. Far more collaboration among nations internationally and within nations such as the United States is therefore needed.

There is also a need for international collaboration on making drug therapies available, especially for HIV/AIDS and certain other diseases. The largest pharmaceutical houses are all multinationals, which should facilitate accomplishment of this goal. Congress, through immigration and welfare reforms in 1996 and a clear demonstration of political fear, said that states were no longer required to provide health care to any legal immigrant who arrived after 1996 but gave the states the option to do so. Several of the most immigrant-rich states, including California and New Jersey, have been providing Medicaid coverage for legal immigrants who arrived after 1996. New York State's supreme court ruled in 2001 that New York's practice of barring legal immigrants from receiving Medicaid violates both the state constitution and the equal protection clause of the U.S. Constitution (Miller, 2001). The National Law Health Program indicated that the case was successful because of a provision in the state constitution that requires New York to provide aid to its poor. This is a trend that bears watching, as lawsuits in other states are expected to follow.

Partnerships: Communities, Government, and Private Stakeholders

Partnerships have been a constant within the health care system for the past hundred years, and they exist in almost every sector and level of the system. Recently, two new forms of partnership have begun to emerge: between CBHOs and managed care companies and between CBHOs and hospitals. This trend holds much promise for the future of U.S. health care systems and for health care service delivery.

CBHO–Managed Care Company Partnerships

Partnerships between CBHOs and managed care (MC) companies are a new and promising trend that is expected to contribute to improved health care services for special populations, including women and children, the poor, and immigrants. As pressure increases for MC and Medicaid Managed Care (MMC) companies to provide evidence of improved outcomes for the populations in their care, they are now seeking assistance to meet this challenge.

One of the entities in the health care environment that managed care companies have turned to is CBHOs.

The CBHO-MC partnership can be mutually beneficial, but it must be structured in ways that are fair and equitable. Therefore, CBHOs have to approach negotiations from a position of strength, which comes from feeling empowered. Empowered CBHOs are very clear about what they want from the partnership, for example:

- Agreement among partners to facilitate community involvement and participation in the program design of services to be delivered
- Strong awareness that a CBHO's knowledge of community is a valuable asset
- Willingness to compensate CBHOs adequately for using their connections to community
- Community feedback used to improve service delivery
- CBHO connection of community to care its members identify and want

The partnerships between CBHOs and MC companies are essentially private business arrangements that are not likely to involve government. If the managed care company serves a Medicaid population, the company does receive government funds, in which case the MC entity can subcontract with a CBHO to provide distinct kinds of services, including outreach, education, counseling (at the individual, peer, or group level), and case management. Most often the MC entity will want to establish a contractual agreement for these services from the CBHO for which the company will pay a nominal per-patient fee for a number of patients in its plan. These are labor-intensive and therefore costly services. Consequently, CBHOs are strongly advised to conduct unit cost analysis of the services they will offer and carefully assess if the amount of the contract will carry the program. CBHOs are urged to obtain financial and legal advice prior to entering into any contractual agreement with a business partner.

CBHO-Hospital Partnerships

Even though many of the large hospitals in the inner cities of the United States sit in the middle of poor communities of color that consist of large numbers of uninsured residents and immigrants, the hospitals did not always regard these communities as the primary client pool to be served. Community residents, for their part, are usually aware of how they are perceived by hospital staff and providers. As a result, there are prestigious medical centers in inner-city areas surrounded by residents who do not regard them as a health care or preventive resource and will only use them when an emergency arises.

The failure to build relationships with surrounding communities has created serious problems for some hospitals in the present turbulent health care climate. Hospital stays continue to shorten, and the entire health system is moving toward a prevention health care model that is community-based. Inpatient hospitals have had no choice but to enter into the highly competitive arena of ambulatory care, but as they moved in this direction, relationships between providers and patients were also changing. Informed health care consumers are demanding greater attention to their overall health than doctors have customarily had to give, and empowered communities are insisting on having greater input into the design and delivery of services. What is more, these trends are projected to intensify as time goes on.

Changes in patient-provider relationships are among the many changes hospitals are confronting as they make the leap to outpatient care without having cultivated relationships with the community for whom they must now attempt to deliver primary and preventive care. CBHOs, particularly those that do not provide clinical care, which is to say that they are not competitors of hospitals, are in a unique position to develop partnerships with hospitals using an innovative concept known as "one-stop shopping."

The One-Stop Shop

This health service concept was developed more than two decades ago to facilitate provision of comprehensive services to underserved populations. The idea behind the one-stop shop is to provide multiple services in one geographical location. Those services should include the full spectrum of primary preventive health services, mental health care, social and support services, immigration services, language services for all groups served, and dental and case management services.

The theory behind one-stop services is that if multiple services identified by a community are provided in one easily accessible location, at convenient times, and in culturally and linguistically sensitive ways, that combination is likely to increase the use of services while also leading to improved health outcomes. CBHOs are integral to the process of creating a one-stop shop, which often means developing a partnership in which a CBHO and a hospital will share space, patients, and other resources. Needless to say, the details and intricacies surrounding service delivery, responsibilities, monitoring, evaluation, and other aspects of the collaboration will have to be carefully negotiated and decided on with the help of legal counsel.

Building and Maintaining Partnerships

The objective of all CBHO partnerships is to improve health and empower community. Nevertheless, the process of developing partnerships or coalitions will depend on what kinds of services the groups are coming together to provide and who these groups are. The kinds of partnerships described in this chapter are presented without regard to their degree of economic success or performance effectiveness. Rather they are meant as examples of win-win partnerships that CBHOs and their partners might negotiate and build in order to meet their common objectives.

The Contra Costa County (California) Health Services Department Prevention Program put together a guide to building and maintaining effective coalitions that has been shared with a wide range of health coalitions (Cohen, Baer, and Satterwhite, 1994). The ideas presented in the guide are an outgrowth of a Special Project of Regional and National Significance (SPRANS) grant awarded to the Contra Costa County Health Services Department by the U.S. Department of Health and Human Services' Maternal and Child Health Division. Most of it has been applied here to building and maintaining CBHO partnerships.

Five Steps to Building Effective Partnerships

1. Analyze the partnership's objectives; assess community strengths and weaknesses; obtain community input regarding its needs; clarify terminology; define the partnership clearly in terms of purpose, mission, and structure, and be certain that both par-

ties understand and agree with the definitions; then determine if both parties want to go ahead with building a partnership.
2. Recruit the right people.
3. Devise both short- and long-term objectives.
4. Anticipate the necessary resources.
5. Define elements of a successful partnership structure, including operating locations, decision-making methods, areas of responsibility, structure of meetings, and conflict management methods.

Two Steps to Maintaining Effective Partnerships

1. Maintain partnership vitality and enthusiasm by addressing any difficulties in the partnership, sharing the power and leadership, providing retreats and training opportunities to deal with the frustrations and exhaustion of partnership work, and celebrating the successes.
2. Conduct evaluation, obtain community input, and use both to make improvements.

Improving Health Outcomes for Everyone

The most important work for poor people in the United States at this time is to safeguard and improve their health. Given the lack of supports, this will be an extremely difficult task to accomplish. Medicaid cuts continue under the present administration and are expected to continue. There are no items on federal or state political agendas at the moment that attempt to address the need to provide coverage for the ever-increasing numbers of uninsured. Legal immigrants continue to struggle for inclusion in health care benefits provided by the state in which they reside, and undocumented immigrants ignore symptoms of poor health in an effort to remain under the radar screen of the immigration services.

Conclusion

Difficult times notwithstanding, CBHOs continue to provide a wide array of health and health-related services that address whole lives and the health needs of whole communities. This book is intended to provide a road map for CBHOs not only to survive but also to thrive as they continue to improve community health through the combined effects of health services and community empowerment.

There is every indication that CBHOs are rising to meet the challenge of providing culturally and linguistically appropriate services to poor communities where mainstream services are either unavailable or inaccessible. While CBHOs have indeed met that challenge and continue to remain focused on those tasks, much hard work remains. There must be a redoubling of emphasis on improving health outcomes. Outcomes are the combined result of patient satisfaction, efficacy, and cost-effectiveness. Patient involvement and participation ensure patient satisfaction and service utilization. However, continued survival dictates that CBHOs now focus their attention on proving their efficacy and cost-effectiveness. To that end, CBHOs will do well to use their advocacy and community-building skills to invite both public and private funding sources into partnerships that will help CBHOs build capacity to collect, analyze, and disseminate data. At this juncture in their history, CBHOs cannot, must not, and we predict will not fail to provide evidence of their role in improving health outcomes and their contributions to community empowerment and development.

Key Points

- Conservative views on social and health policy contribute to a climate of dwindling resources to support the work of CBHOs.
- CBHOs in poor communities are at the center in educating their clients and organizing them to seek health care resources.
- Ongoing changes in U.S. health care and persistent health disparities provide opportunities that CBHOs must use to demonstrate the significant work that they do.
- New research and science are transforming the U.S. health care delivery system.
- Adult education practices in the international community hold promise for work with low-income communities here in the United States.
- Shifting theoretical perspectives are moving the United States toward prevention, health promotion, and primary care as prime modalities for health service delivery.

- Community organizing, building, and empowerment are critical to improving health outcomes.
- Two community empowerment models, the Freire model and the CBHO intervention model, hold great promise for community change and community health.
- CBHO partnerships with managed care companies, with hospitals, and as one-stop entities are projected to increase.

Study Questions

1. As noted in this chapter, the United States currently faces ten health care challenges. Select one of these challenges, and investigate the national efforts in place to address it. Then apply what is being done nationally to how the problem has affected low-income members of a community in your city, and provide an analysis of how effective the national program is in your local community.

2. You are the executive director of a CBHO in your city. One of your largest grants is for HIV/AIDS counseling and support services. You were notified of this grant eight months ago by your local department of health and were told to start up services. You hired twelve social workers who provide in-depth case management services to a combined caseload of approximately 750 people, including HIV/AIDS clients and their families. Your agency is one of five in the city that received notifications of this grant award, but neither your agency nor any of the others have received any monies to date. Develop a plan to build and maintain an HIV/AIDS coalition that will be empowered enough to advocate with the city for resources to provide services to your HIV/AIDS clients and their families.

References

Alexander, J., Nank, R., and Stivers, C. "Implications of Welfare Reform: Do Nonprofit Survival Strategies Threaten Civil Society?" *Nonprofit and Voluntary Sector Quarterly*, 1999, *28*, 452–475.

Austin, J. E. "Strategic Collaboration Between Nonprofits and Businesses." *Nonprofit and Voluntary Sector Quarterly*, 2000, *29*, 69–97.

Bayne Smith, M. A. "Primary Care Choices and Opportunities for Racial/Ethnic Minority Populations in the USA and UK: A Comparative Analysis." *Ethnicity and Health*, 1999, *4*, 165–188.

Bayne Smith, M. A. "Promoting Heart Disease Prevention at Work Sites in Queens, New York City." Paper presented at the sixteenth National Conference on Chronic Disease Prevention and Control, Atlanta, Mar. 2002.

Bayne Smith, M. A., and Perot, R. *Report of Environmental Scan of Consumer Advocacy Needs and Requirements in the District of Columbia.* Washington, D.C.: Consumer Health Foundation, 2003.

Bayne Smith, M. A., and others. "Improvements in Heart Health Behaviors and Reduction in Coronary Artery Disease Risk Factors in Urban Teenage Females Through School-Based Intervention: The PATH Program." *American Journal of Public Health,* 2004, *94,* 1538–1543.

Beito, D. T. "Poor Before Welfare." *National Review,* May 6, 1996, pp. 42–44.

Bruce, T. A., McKane, S. U., and Brock, R. M. "Taking a Community-Based Public Health Approach: How Does It Make a Difference?" In T. A. Bruce and S. U. McKane (eds.), *Community-Based Public Health: A Partnership Model.* Washington, D.C.: American Public Health Association, 2000.

Brundtland, G. H. *The World Health Report, 2002: Reducing Risks, Promoting Healthy Life.* Geneva: World Health Organization, 2002.

Carroll, T. *Intermediary NGOs: The Supporting Link in Grassroots Development.* Bloomfield, Conn.: Kumarian Press, 1992.

Center on Budget and Policy Priorities. "Census Data Show Poverty Increased, Income Stagnated, and the Number of Uninsured Rose to a Record Level in 2003." Press release. Washington, D.C.: Center on Budget and Policy Priorities, Aug. 27, 2004.

Clark-Amankwaa, L. "Post Partum Depression, Culture, and African-American Women." *Journal of Cultural Diversity,* 2003, *24,* 297–316.

Cohen, J. E. *Politics and Economic Policy in the United States.* (2nd ed.) New York: Houghton Mifflin, 2000.

Cohen, L., Baer, N., and Satterwhite, P. *Developing Effective Coalitions: An Eight-Step Guide.* Martinez, Calif.: Contra Costa County Health Services Department Prevention Program, 1994.

"Community Programs Can Help Reduce Rates of Heart Disease." *Heart Disease Weekly,* July 2, 2000, p. 7.

Cornachio, D. "An Interview with Katherine Newman—Running in Place: Can People Still Work Their Way out of Poverty?" *Ford Foundation Report,* 2003, *34*(3), 21–23.

Delgado, D. Y. *Plain Talk/Hablando Claro: What Works to Reduce Pregnancy, STDs, and HIV/AIDS for African American and Latino Youth.* Paper presented at the NOAPPP Pre-Conference Institute, Arlington, Va., Nov. 2003.

Edwards, E. D., and Egbert-Edwards, M. "Community Development with American Indians and Alaska Natives." In F. G. Rivera and J. L. Erlich (eds.), *Community Organizing in a Diverse Society.* Boston: Allyn & Bacon, 1998.

Ehrenreich, B., and English, D. *Complaints and Disorders: The Sexual Politics of Sickness.* New York: Feminist Press, City University of New York, 1973.

Fisher, K. J., and others. "Organizational Characteristics Associated with Smokeless Tobacco Use." *Health Values,* 1994, *18*(4), 34–40.

Forrest, C. B., and Whelan, E. M. "Primary Care Safety Net Delivery Sites in the United States: A Comparison of Community Health Centers, Hospital Outpatient Departments, and Physician Offices." *Journal of the American Medical Association,* 2000, *284*, 2077–2083.

Fredericksen, P., and London, R. "Disconnect in the Hollow State: The Pivotal Role of Organizational Capacity in Community-Based Development Organizations." *Public Administration Review,* 2000, *60*, 230–239.

Freire, P. *Pedagogy of the Oppressed.* New York: Continuum, 1990.

Galjart, B. "Counter-Development: Possibilities and Constraints." In G. Craig and M. Mayo (eds.), *Community Empowerment: A Reader in Participation and Development.* London: Zed Books, 1995.

Gergen, D. "To Have and to Have Less." *U. S. News and World Report,* July 26, 1999, p. 64.

Gordon, G. "Participation, Empowerment and Sexual Health in Africa." In G. Craig and M. Mayo (eds.), *Community Empowerment: A Reader in Participation and Development.* London: Zed Books, 1995.

Green, R. H. "Politics, Power and Poverty: Health for All in 2000 in the Third World." *Social Science and Medicine,* 1991, *32*, 745–755.

Greenhouse, S. "Immigrants Rally in City, Seeking Rights." *New York Times,* Oct. 5, 2003, p. 33.

Grossman, J. B., Walker, K. E., Kotloff, L. J., and Pepper, S. *Adult Communication and Teen Sex: Changing a Community.* Philadelphia: Public/Private Ventures, 2001.

Guiden, M. "Health Care Hurt by Medicaid Cuts: Millions Could Be Affected." *Focus,* Nov.-Dec. 2002, p. 12.

Halpern, R. *Rebuilding the Inner City: A History of Neighborhood Initiatives to Address Poverty in the United States.* New York: Columbia University Press, 1995.

Heckler, M. M. *Report of the Secretary's Task Force on Black and Minority Health,* Vol. 2: *Crosscutting Issues in Minority Health.* Washington, D.C.: U.S. Department of Health and Human Services, 1985.

Hood, J. "Take Your Medicine." *National Review,* June 30, 2003, pp. 27–28.

Irigoyen, M., and Findley, S. E. "Methodological Difficulties in Assessing

Contributions by Community-Based Organizations to Improving Child Health." Editorial. *Archives of Pediatric and Adolescent Medicine*, 1998, *152*, 318–320.

Kaufman, J., and Joseph-Fox, Y. K. "American Indian and Alaska Native Women." In M. Bayne-Smith (ed.), *Race, Gender, and Health*. Thousand Oaks, Calif.: Sage, 1996.

Kegeles, S. D., Hays, R. B., and Coates, T. J. "The Mpowerment Project: A Community-Level HIV Prevention Intervention for Young Gay Men." *American Journal of Public Health*, 1996, *86*, 1129–1136.

Kelly, J. A., Saint Lawrence, J. S., and Stevenson, L. Y. "Community AIDS/HIV Risk Reduction: The Effects of Endorsement by Popular People in Three Cities." *American Journal of Public Health*, 1992, *82*, 1483–1489.

Koplan, J. P., and Fleming, D. W. "Current and Future Public Health Challenges." *Journal of the American Medical Association*, 2000, *284*, 1696–1698.

Kreuter, M. W. "PATCH: Its Origin, Basic Concepts, and Links to Contemporary Public Health Policy." *Journal of Health Education*, 1992, *23*, 135–139.

Kreuter, M. W., Lezin, N. A., Kreuter, M. W., and Green, L. W. *Community Health Promotion Ideas That Work*. (2nd ed.) Boston: Jones & Bartlett, 2003.

LaVeist, T. A. "The Political Empowerment and Health Status of African Americans: Mapping a New Territory." *American Journal of Sociology*, 1992, *97*(4), 1080–1095.

Leonhardt, D. "Employment Rises for the First Time in Seven Months." *New York Times*, Oct. 4, 2003, p. A1.

Liebschutz, S. E. "Coping by Nonprofit Organizations During the Reagan Years." *Nonprofit Management and Leadership*, 1992, *2*, 363–380.

Mattessich, P., and Monsey, B. *Community Building: What Makes It Work—A Review of Factors Influencing Successful Building*. Saint Paul, Minn.: Wilder Research Center, 2001.

Mayo, M., and Craig, G. "Increasing Community Participation and Empowerment." In G. Craig and M. Mayo (eds.), *Community Empowerment: A Reader in Participation and Development*. London: Zed Books, 1995.

McBride, D. "Black America: From Community Health Care to Crisis Medicine." In J. A. Morone and G. S. Belkin (eds.), *The Politics of Health Care Reform: Lessons from the Past, Prospects for the Future*. Durham, N.C.: Duke University Press, 1994.

McKnight, J. L. "Rationale for a Community Approach to Health Improvement." In T. A. Bruce and S. U. McKane (eds.), *Community-Based Public Health: A Partnership Model*. Washington, D.C.: American

Public Health Association, 2000.

Miller, S. B. "Immigrant Healthcare: Must States Cover Cost?" *Christian Science Monitor,* June 13, 2001, p. 1.

Minkler, M., and Wallerstein, N. "Improving Health Through Community Organizing and Community Building." In M. Minkler (ed.), *Community Organizing and Community Building for Health.* New Brunswick, N.J.: Rutgers University Press, 2002.

Morrison, J. D., and others. "Strengthening Neighborhoods by Developing Community Networks." *Social Work,* 1997, *42,* 527–535.

New York City Department of Health and Mental Hygiene. *Health Disparities in New York City.* New York City: Commonwealth Fund, 2004.

O'Gorman, F. "Brazilian Community Development: Changes and Challenges." In G. Craig and M. Mayo (eds.), *Community Empowerment: A Reader in Participation and Development.* London: Zed Books, 1995.

O'Neil, E. H. *Health Professions Education for the Future: Schools in Service to the Nation.* San Francisco: Pew Health Professions Commission, 1993.

Proschaska, J. L., and Velicer, W. F. "The Transtheoretical Model of Health Behavior Change." *American Journal of Health Promotion,* 1997, *12,* 38–48.

Putnam, R. "The Strange Disappearance of Civic America." *American Prospect,* 1996, *24,* 34–38.

Randall-David, E. *Strategies for Working with Culturally Diverse Communities and Clients.* Washington, D.C.: Association for the Care of Children's Health, 1989.

Rivera, F. G., and Erlich, J. L. "Epilogue: The Twenty-First Century—Promise or Illusion?" In F. G. Rivera and J. L. Erlich (eds.), *Community Organizing in a Diverse Society.* Boston: Allyn & Bacon, 1998.

Rosenberg, G. "Challenges of Managed Care for Health Professionals: Implications for Social Work Practice." In A. Katz, A. Lurie, and C. Vidal (eds.), *Critical Social Welfare Issues: Tools for Social Work and Health Care Professionals.* Binghamton, N.Y.: Haworth Press, 1997.

Schacht, J. "Creating Partnerships with Clinic Associations to Preserve the Safety Net: Evaluation Report." *Health Affairs,* 1998, *17*(3), 1–5.

Schauffler, H. H., and Wolin, J. "Community Health Clinics Under Managed Care Competition: Navigating Uncharted Waters." *Journal of Health Politics, Policy and Law,* 1996, *21,* 461–488.

Speak, S. "Children in Urban Regeneration: Foundations for Sustainable Participation." *Community Development Journal,* 2000, *35,* 31–40.

Withorn, A., and Jons, P. *Worrying About Welfare Reform: Community-Based Agencies Respond.* Boston: Boston Area Academics Working Group on Poverty, 1999.

The Authors

Marcia Bayne Smith is associate professor of urban studies at Queens College, City University of New York. She has conducted research and published extensively on the health issues of women, immigrants, and racial and ethnic minorities. Her work has appeared in the *Journal of Health Education,* the *Journal of Community Practice, Research in Social Policy, The Encyclopedia of New York City,* the *Journal of Cardiopulmonary Rehabilitation,* the *American Journal of Public Health,* and the *International Journal of Ethnicity and Health.* She served as editor and contributing author of the book *Race, Gender, and Health* (Sage, 1996), which focuses on the health status of four different groups of women (Native Americans and Alaska Natives, African Americans, Asians and Pacific Islanders, and Hispanics) and their relationships with the Western-based U.S. health care system.

A ceaseless worker on behalf of the community, Bayne-Smith has recently completed a ten-year stint as the chair of the board of directors of the Caribbean Women's Health Association, Inc.(CWHA). During her tenure, CWHA's growth has remained focused on community needs. Toward that end, CWHA, in partnership with Lutheran Medical Center and the Sunset Park Family Health Care Network, completed development of the Caribbean-American Family Health Center (CAFHC), acknowledged as a national "Center of Excellence" by the U.S. Department of Health and Human Services. Bayne Smith, who also sits on the board of the Public Health Association of New York City, holds a doctorate in social welfare with a concentration in health care policy from Columbia University's School of Social Welfare.

Yvonne J. Graham, Brooklyn's deputy borough president, has been a pioneer in the area of public health for more than two decades. She is the founder and former executive director of the Caribbean

Women's Health Association, Inc. (CWHA), which provides comprehensive culturally sensitive health care, immigration, social, and support services to a diverse constituency. Graham is a registered nurse and holds a master's degree in public health from Hunter College at the City University of New York (CUNY).

As Brooklyn's deputy borough president, Graham oversees health care policy, public education policy, social services, and constituent services. Brooklyn is one of the largest employers of health care workers and professionals in the state of New York, and Graham uses her experience working with immigrants, community activists, academics, and elected officials to serve as a powerful advocate for Brooklyn's ninety-three different ethnic groups.

Graham is currently a member of Hunter College, the CUNY external advisory committee, the advisory committee of the School of Nursing at Long Island University, the foundation board of Kingsborough Community College, and the President's Community Council at Brooklyn College.

She has been the recipient of numerous awards, including the National Public Citizen of the Year Award from the National Association of Black Social Workers.

Sally Guttmacher has conducted community-based research for a number of years. Her doctorate from the Division of Sociomedical Sciences at Columbia University reflects her academic background in anthropology, sociology, and public health. She is the director of the master's in public health program at New York University. Guttmacher's interests are in social epidemiology, reproductive health, and community-based interventions and evaluation.

She is a past president and current board member of the Public Health Association of New York City and a past chair of the Medical Care Section of the American Public Health Association, where she serves on the governing council. She is also a member of the board of the Caribbean Women's Health Association, Inc., and a fellow of the Master Scholars Program at the New York University Medical School. She has recently been selected as a senior Fulbright scholar.

Name Index

Subject Index